Towards a
SOULFUL SEXUALITY

by

Adele Gruber

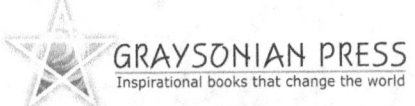

GRAYSONIAN PRESS
Inspirational books that change the world

Copyright © 2007, 2011 Adele Gruber
All rights reserved under international copyright conventions.

First published (2007) under the name Hanna G Ruby by Booksurge. (ISBN 978-1419676819)

Published 2011 by Graysonian Press

No part of this book may be reproduced, stored in a retrieval system, or transmitted in any form or by any means electronic, mechanical, photocopying, recorded

Printed in Australia 2012

Whilst every care has been taken to check the accuracy of the information in this book, the publisher cannot be held responsible for any errors, omissions or originality.
ISBN: 978-0-620-46120-7

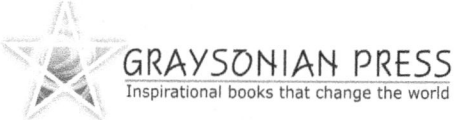

GRAYSONIAN PRESS
Inspirational books that change the world

www.graysonian.com   pat@graysonian.com

Book designed by Rachel Brown
indigoconcepts@gmail.com

Towards a SOULFUL SEXUALITY

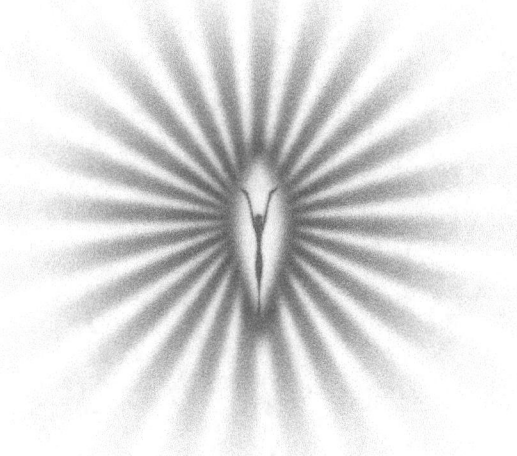

NEW PERSPECTIVES OF SEX, AGE AND MENOPAUSE
FOR WOMEN 35 TO 60 PLUS

Adele Gruber

PREFACE

This book is called Towards a Sacred Sexuality because it is an initial step in the direction of a destination towards which I believe we should journey. This is a renewed consciousness of a feminine sexual holiness firmly grounded in our bodies and our psyches that should apply throughout a women's life, even, and most especially, in the post-menopausal years.

The first steps must be to know why you should take the journey at all. For this I offer my Manifesto that informs and explains the cultural, historical background to our deep ambivalences around these matters. It attempts to separate fact from fiction regarding the nature of sex, love and spirituality, women's sexual anatomy and the concept (and history) of menopause & aging.

This book represents my sincere attempt to work towards a soulful sexuality. To start with, we are required to review, redefine and re-imagine our core beliefs and feelings around these subjects. The Manifesto incorporates three condensed histories full of intriguing facts:

- past perceptions of menopause and stereotypes of aging women
- the history of female sexual anatomy, modern Western sexology and Eastern esoteric secrets
- and overviews the essential nature of sex, from the physical to the metaphysical, to challenge your core beliefs about body, mind, spirit – and sex.

I then encourage you to re-examine your own sexuality and be prepared to heal your deepest psychic wounds. In this respect I offer a short Self-Assessment Questionnaire so that you can review your sexual self to determine how "clear" you may be on sexual issues?

The Healing Workbook "Working with my Sexuality" is a personal program of reflections, memories, exercises and meditations that will enable you to better understand your own personal patterns and history around the issues raised in the Manifesto.

Having read the Manifesto and completed the Healing Workbook, you can say at best, that you are en route to or on the way towards to a more soulful sexuality. There is much more to read, personal issues to heal, techniques to learn, meditations to practice and awareness to raise, wisdoms to internalize.

It is still a field being uncovered by psychologists, spiritual teachers, body practitioners, sexologists and others.

I hope you enjoy your journey towards…

CONTENTS

PART ONE
MANIFESTO: Sex, Age & Menopause

CHAPTER ONE
Sexual Dichotomies

- 1.1 A deeply divided legacy 4
- 1.2 When sex becomes dirty 7
- 1.3 Post-menopausal challenge of the new millenium 10
- 1.4 Fear of ageing - fear and sex 14

CHAPTER TWO
"Old" Menopause & Beyond

- 2.1 Ill omens and ghost images 20
- 2.2 Bloodlettings, dark humours & witches 22
- 2.3 Submissions & Sublimination; the good wife and grandmother 25
- 2.4 Vital ageing, reform & Sarah Bernhardt 27
- 2.5 Medicalized, pathologized & psychoanalyzed 30
- 2.6 Another kind of menopause 36

CHAPTER THREE
Sexual Anatomy as Destiny

- 3.1 A destiny of inferior organs 42
- 3.2 Love my Yoni, love myself 45
- 3.3 Eve's secrets of vagina 101 48
- 3.4 No longer passive plumbing 51
- 3.5 Our "hysterical" travelling uterus 53
- 3.6 Orgasm and ejaculation 57

CHAPTER FOUR
Sex: Sacred & Profane

- 4.1 Human sex is 66
- 4.2 The basics (including the bad, sad & dutiful) 69
- 4.3 Sacred ceremony & ritual union 76
- 4.4 Vitality, health and longevity 81
- 4.5 Eros and ecstasy: getting high on sex 83
- 4.6 Cosmic energy & quantum sex 86

CHAPTER FIVE
Towards a new "old" age

- 5.1 Goddess metaphors & the Hekate problem 94
- 5.2 Reclaiming the crone 100
- 5.3 Living in a quantum world 105
- 5.4 Death, ageing and sexual beauty 108
- 5.5 Life ongoing 114

Appendix 117

PART TWO
SELF-ASSESSMENT QUESTIONAIRE
Review your sexual self 120

PART THREE
HEALING WORKBOOK
Working with my Sexuality

1. Uncovering Core Beliefs 125
2. Recalling Sexual History 130
3. Meeting Body & Soul 132
4. Making new choices 135

Biography 142

Endnotes 145

PART ONE

MANIFESTO:
Sex, Age & Menopause

CHAPTER 1
SEXUAL DICHOTOMIES

She is wise: she is witch
She is spiritual: she is material
She is asexual; or dangerously sexual
She is benign and useless: ugly and evil
She is the good aunt, grandmother, or activist
Or the evil stepmother; and old hag who
keeps princesses locked in towers.

1.1 A DEEPLY DIVIDED LEGACY

Deep dichotomies in the perception of older women run like fault lines through our culture, confusing and confining us.

Women in general have been defined by their sexuality – or at least by the prevailing "scientific" understanding of that sexuality. Conflicting viewpoints recur endlessly: women were idealized, or derided; revered, or reviled as evil, messy matter – inherently bad, inferior, or banal at best.

The matter of the ageing feminine is worse; images of witches, ugliness, and uselessness. The duality, the dichotomy of good and evil, is ever present in the evaluation of women in general, and older women in particular. When they are good, they are very, very good, and when they are bad, they are sexual!

The duality is primeval; as reflected in these words from an ancient mysterious female oracle:

> *For I am the first and the last,*
> *I am the honoured one and the scorned one*
> *I am the whore and the holy one.*
> *I am the wife and the virgin.*[1]

"Within Western experience lies a long legacy of denigrating ageing women, especially in their postmenopausal years," writes Louis Banner.[2] Older women generally had a very hard time: only

---

Women in general have been defined by their sexuality – or at least by the prevailing "scientific" understanding of that sexuality.

the authority of money, class, or political clout lessened the sting. They were considered in league with the devil (sorcery and witchcraft were always connected to older women), or in the clutch of a deep pathology – menopause and old age as illness, madness, or, at least, a deficiency of sorts.

Contradictory theories abound; older women were not supposed to have sexual feelings, or else they had too many and needed to be controlled. "The whole of woman is sex," insists an old Latin proverb.[3]

On the other hand ... "The majority of women (happily for them) are not very much troubled with sexual feelings of any kind. What men are habitually, women are only exceptionally," wrote a medical authority of the 1850s.[4]

We, the baby boomers, were born into a world with another version of this dichotomy: we could be respectable (meaning a virgin before marriage and sexually passive as wife), or we could choose to be a "besmirched, worldly woman who enjoyed sex".[5] The 1960s sexual revolution exploded these restricted sexual options.

But freshly unplugged repression is still rebellious, adolescent, uncontained. We knew what we were being liberated from – or so we thought. Oral contraception, legalized abortion and the focus on female orgasm supported a drastic break from the past. But the sense of freedom held illusions as well. Sex without consequence was a liberty of sorts; but still masculine in nature. There was no essential

---

But freshly unplugged repression is still rebellious, adolescent, uncontained. We knew what we were being liberated from – or so we thought.

feminine sensibility to imbue this liberation with consciousness of a different order.

Opposition to restrictive values is not enough; we must be FOR something valuable as well. The initial unbridled enthusiasm faltered in mindless swinging; it never really matured nor found a link to an alternate universe of value and meaning. Without such a container, the momentum stalled. The rise of fundamentalist religion facilitated an overt return to the certainties of the old morality for many, reinforced by fear of the Aids pandemic which began in the 1980s.

Now that the children of the swinging 1960s are approaching their own 60s, the sexual challenge renews itself in a different way. What kind of sexuality is relevant now – if any at all? So many seem to be embracing – or resigning themselves to – an asexual old age; not only becoming sexually inactive because there might be no one to "have sex" with, but by switching off the living active awareness of sexual energy in their lives.

"Sexually active" and an active sexuality are confused.

Now that the children of the swinging 1960s are approaching their own 60s, the sexual challenge renews itself in a different way. What kind of sexuality is relevant now - if any at all?

1.2 WHEN SEX BECAME DIRTY

Once upon a time sex was enjoyed without shame, as a gift of God, Goddess, the Great Spirit – an act of joy, of devotion, something perfectly natural and wholly divine – all at the same time.

Once upon a time the goddesses were venerated as the embodiment of love, passion, and sex, which were considered holy when performed in reverence for and in service of the female divinity.

But the mindset of patriarchy killed off the Goddess more than five thousand years ago. She was constrained to submission at worst, or virginal purity and celibacy at best; her divinity denied. With that, the idea of sexuality as spirituality, as something inherently divine, was eradicated for all women – young and old. Indeed, for all men as well!

Sexuality was severed from spirituality and became its extreme opposite; sex was dirty, primitive, and instinctual (and feminine in nature), while spirituality was pure and clean and transcendent (and masculine in nature).

In the West, however, it was only from our Bible onwards that sexuality became a sin, the means by which the devil could tempt mankind into damnation, a shameful necessity of physical gratification that was obscene and dirty. Only from our Bible onwards, were women considered inherently sinful and destined for eternal punishment.

Only from our Bible onwards, were women considered inherently sinful and destined for eternal punishment.

Even before Eve bit that apple, there was poor, feisty Lilith (born initially as one with Adam – "male and female created He them" says the first Biblical reference), who, according to legend, preferred to have sex on top. Lilith represents lunar consciousness (waxing and waning, death and rebirth), sexuality, body, and intuitive wisdom – all of which patriarchy degraded and denied. She got a terribly bad press.

Previously, the Goddess had ruled the mysteries of sexuality, birth, life, and death. Now the patriarchal God took control of life and death, and split procreation and motherhood from sexuality and "magic and mystery". Lilith refused to submit and flew off in a rage. Until recent decades, she has been universally demonized as seductive, witch, outcast – the enraged, avenging goddess, wife of Satan.

Solar was split from lunar; psyche from soma or physical, corresponding to a general disassociation from the body. Mind and body, spirit and body, soul and body were split entities, and unequal. The body was inferior, an unfortunate necessity – together with its most basic of functions, sex; and it was associated with the feminine. (I once read an old text that described women as "bags of filth". The males' organs of excretion were not referred to.)

Male and female were unequal; spirit and nature were unequal. Man headed the chain of command – after God. As women, and as a culture, we have paid dearly for this division. The misogyny of the patriarchy affected all cultures in the last 2000 years, one way or another.

Mind and body, spirit and body, soul and body were split entities, and unequal. The body was inferior, an unfortunate necessity ...

The fierce, sexual, independent-spirited wise dark goddess aspect of Lilith was replaced by submissive Eve, who was yet blamed for the whole messy business anyway. She was the sinful one, secondary to Adam, and cursed forever to give birth in pain. (Medieval midwives were sinning when they alleviated the pain of childbirth.)

As long as Eve is sinful and physical matter corrupt in any way whatsoever, our sexuality is compromized – and our liberation incomplete. This split must be healed.

I am proposing that sexuality and spirituality are aspects of the same thing; that the split between psyche and soma (the physical) is resolved in the energetic unity of a higher order. "We have lost contact with what unites them," says Alexander Lowen in The Spirituality of the Body.[6] Sexuality is psychosomatic – and by that I mean, not that it's some kind of illness, in the more common meaning of the word, but that it overtly operates on both the physical and the psychic level.

Where science and religion are finding rapprochement in the infinite wave world of quantum physics, we find fresh metaphors for the lost unifying element. Waves of sexual sensations that emanate from the body can be visualized as cosmic, psychic energy, high-frequency vibrations that bridge us to higher consciousness.

These metaphors indicate possibilities that have profound implications generally, and more so for you and me now, as ageing women today.

The fierce, sexual, independent-spirited wise dark goddess aspect of Lilith was replaced by submissive Eve, who was yet blamed for the whole messy business anyway.

1.3 POST-MENOPAUSAL CHALLENGE OF THE NEW MILLENNIUM

Female baby boomers are well into menopause – and beyond; part of a giant wave of grey (even though the grey has been tinted somewhat).

There are more woman over the age of 50 in the world today than probably ever before in history; 45 million US women born in the baby boom years alone are now doing the critical menopause passage, and 11 million UK women. Globally, age distribution in the older category is increasing in all the more developed countries.

"One of the blessings of being part of that enormous wave of women moving past age fifty today is that we are more authoritative, assertive and self assured than any generation of menopausal women before us. And we have more economic power," writes feminist author Nancy Friday.[7] (She was controversial among feminists for proclaiming feminism and appreciating men and sex. They were for her not mutually exclusive.)

Nevertheless, there seems to be a pronounced loss of confidence as age advances. Death might or might not scare us, but ageing confuses and confounds us so! The old stereotypes won't do; but they haunt us still – especially sexually.

Why is it that so many of my contemporaries who also "did' the 1960s as teenagers or young adults, and spent the last 40 plus years as modern women applying dedication and commitment to their

---

Female baby boomers are well into menopause – and beyond; part of a giant wave of grey (even though the grey has been tinted somewhat).

homes, families, and work, are now faltering and wilting as they approach their 60s? Without admirable models of being post-menopausal in our time, the once feisty, wobble.

Menopause is a transitional experience leading to the rest of our lives. And it's this "rest of our life" we need to reinvent. I would like to think that as we baby boomers enter the other side of 50 with a reasonable lifespan and quality of life ahead we can redefine ageing – and sexuality.

Statistically, we have a chunk of good years ahead of us. How do we intend to live them?

What have the health advances, new technologies, economic empowerment, psychological process, and spirituality, previously inaccessible to the mainstream, made realistically achievable for us as the "ageing" boomers of the early 21st century?

What is reasonably possible? What is wishful thinking? What is optimum? What is delusional narcissism? That is the question and the challenge. In this new millennium (provided extremism doesn't catapult us into Armageddon), ageing can be different – should be different – and much, much better.

For personal perspective ...

Little more than a hundred years ago, without the advances in medical and eye technology (and the chemistry of hair colour, dare I say),

---

Menopause is a transitional experience leading to the rest of our lives. And it's this "rest of our life" we need to reinvent.

I would probably have been a toothless, blind old "hag" in my mid-fifties, if I was alive at all. My life choices would have been constrained by my plebeian, non-aristocratic status to much onerous duty, since – had I otherwise been who I am today – I would have been no rich Lady of rank.

I am glad to be alive in these times. The ordinary person has so many more options than ever before. No longer living the harsh grind of daily subsistence and inferior legal status, we can look at ourselves as woman over 50 and say – OK, now what? We have the opportunity to live differently. The cliché applies; another new stage has only just begun. Post-menopause and "ageing" is the new frontier.

But first we must disentangle ourselves from the absurd and awful stereotypes of older women, specifically, and sex and ageing in general, that infect our culture – and deeply affect our own self-evaluations. These nasty assumptions define who we become; they are the inevitable facts of our reality. They undermine our courage and our self-image.

We are terrified of becoming ugly old hags. The word hagia, which means "holy" in Greek,[8] was once a reverential title for wise and respected older women; it degraded to "hag". How did the revered and sacred come to mean old and ugly?

Being sexual AFTER the biological time for childbirth is, theoretically, a time of freedom to explore, to enjoy all that sex is and can be. At least we can explore other aspects when we don't have to worry about getting physically pregnant - or not.

We must disentangle ourselves from the absurd and awful stereotypes of older women, specifically, and sex and ageing in general, that infect our culture – and deeply affect our own self-evaluations.

So why is menopause so often the death of sex itself – too ridiculous to contemplate? What is the nature of our current sexuality? Does our mature sexuality embarrass or inspire us, or has menopause killed all interest? Do we want an asexual old age, or do we want to be sexual "forever"?

So why is menopause so often the death of sex itself – too ridiculous to contemplate?

1.4 FEAR OF AGEING - FEAR OF SEX

"Our sexual appetites aren't lost as we age; it is the image of ourselves as sexual that we dutifully abandon to fit the bygone stereotype of patriarchy," says Friday.[9] There are many conflicting stereotypes, and they are all contaminated with a deep-seated fear of ageing, of women – and of sex.

Is old age about progressive, inevitable, inexorable decline, or is old age about living healthily until it is time to pass over; a time of wisdom, joy, and delight? An adventure in evolution!

Attitudes to ageing have themselves changed. And with the health support we have these days, from conventional medicine to alternative healing, our humble earth-suit of flesh and bones in which we navigate this beautiful planet can support a meaningful life for a long time – well, a longer time, for sure.

"Old age can be pitiful and a time for deep regret," says the Indian god Shiva in Sexual Secrets.[10] It can also be "transcendental, glorious, potentially divine".

Deepak Chopra[11] suggests that death by severe illness is the result of a self-fulfilling prophecy with which our culture has indoctrinated us. Yes, we have to pass over some time. But we don't have to get so terribly ill and ail for years in order to die. We can perhaps depart this life, when it's our time, in reasonable health, at senior years – with grace? (Tibetan monks have been doing just that for aeons.)

"Our sexual appetites aren't lost as we age; it is the image of ourselves as sexual that we dutifully abandon to fit the bygone stereotype of patriarchy," says Friday.

It is so easy to ridicule those who try to defy ageing with an obsession with health, exercise, and expensive surgical interventions for face and body. But maybe we are missing something here in our easy cynicism, morbid acceptance – and hidden jealousy.

Between total capitulation to creeping decrepitude and illness, and total obsession with looking/being/becoming narcissistically young, there is a genuine opportunity for living vital, healthy, and meaningful lives, for as long as possible – and then leaving for the other side.

If all the space-age technologies mean anything, it's surely for us to distil some of the cutting-edge gems of health, nutrition, exercise, medical and alternative technologies, and old and modern techniques and attitudes, and use them to live better, longer. (If we can look reasonably good at the same time, why not?)

But the media mock us.

Poor Madonna! Her age-defying exploits attract the best and worst of acerbic public comment, and upstage her art. A tabloid found it newsworthy to describe her left hand as "remarkably bony, wrinkled and covered in protruding veins".[12] Who cares? She can surely dance.

It further praised "her pioneering work on behalf of women of a certain age who refuse to go quietly into the Hush Puppies phase. When we see Madonna, we feel like shouting, 'Oh, give it a rest.' Then again, we dread her hanging up her dance tights, because that means our time will come too." How do we cope with such a deep divide on how we are supposed to age?

... there is a genuine opportunity for living vital, healthy, and meaningful lives, for as long as possible – and then leaving for the other side.

(I love the wonderful irony of her name – as if the controversy surrounding her exploits of personal reinvention parallels the re-imagination of what the Madonna archetype stands for in Western culture.)

We denigrate ourselves – and other older women – with infected attitudes that seep out from the deepest subterranean corridors of consciousness – and unconsciousness. Psychic shadows from down the centuries, and popular culture, wrap themselves around our body, our sex, our beauty, around being female or ageing, and female ageing in particular. Few are impervious. I know that I am not.

Are we succumbing to fear of ageing? Has it become worse, even though we are living longer and longer?

Nancy Friday believes it is so. She relates this psychologically to our fear of going against the sexual condemnation of the "good mother" we have created within ourselves, in whose presence we have split off from all that is associated with the "bad mother". The good girl is good mother's girl, chaste and pure; the bad girl our unacceptable sexual self – the harlot, the one who enjoys sex, the one "good mother" finds hard to love.

As we age, the bad mother comes to haunt us when we look in our mirrors. Are we ageing better than previous generations or not? Do we still perceive ageing as ugly, and old women as repulsive? Do we see reflections of the witch and the evil stepmother of fairy tales, who didn't like the little heroine of the stories?

We denigrate ourselves – and other older women – with infected attitudes that seep out from the deepest subterranean corridors of consciousness – and unconsciousness.

These ubiquitous fairy-tale images of evil old women relate to those "dark" aspects of our mothers that we split off from our conscious self-image – as indeed did she, our real mother (or so, perhaps, it seemed to us), who didn't really like our essential female selves – especially when we touched ourselves – down there.

Although dread of the unacceptable self operates at all ages, it is more ambiguous in our pre-menopausal years, when it is mediated by firm flesh, an overtly celebrated (and exploited) sexual beauty, and our status as mothers, potential mothers, and tax-paying citizens. It just gets so much worse as the mirror image sags somewhat.

This fear, the conflicting personas of ageing women and the endemic contradiction between good and bad sex, has a very long lineage, made worse by an irresolute response to our youth-obsessed age

"Most grim of all," Friday continues, "until we change what was loathsome into something beautiful, which in essence is human sexuality, our children will grow up vulnerable to all the deadly plagues associated with irresponsible sex."[13] Resolving this challenge will also make a sexual older age less absurd and unimaginable; it works both ways. Sex itself needs to be redeemed. And ageing needs to be revisioned.

We are not talking here about a compulsion to stay forever immaturely young. We are talking about a real possibility, in this time, to live long and well, to review what ageing need be. Indeed, what life can be.

We are talking about a real possibility, in this time, to live long and well, to review what ageing need be.

All the strange adjustments of the past, their dysfunctional, neurotic or disturbed motivations, do not alter the fact that today we do not have to go meekly into a decrepit dark night. We can redefine and re-imagine ourselves – and our lives.

But first we must uncover the attitudes and beliefs that linger and lurk in our deepest, darkest unconscious, that yet drive our thoughts, feelings, and actions. They affect our experience of menopause – and our expectations for the rest of our lives.

Come let us excavate the old psychic shadows that haunt us, by examining the stereotypes of post-menopausal women in recent centuries.

After that, we will review our sexual anatomy – just in case we are under the delusion that it has always been properly understood, which it hasn't. Amazingly, we got to the moon before we had a clear science of female sexual anatomy.

Next, we will explore the diverse nature of sexual energy itself. Only then can we dare to imagine other ways of being, and make new choices.

Amazingly, we got to the moon before we had a clear science of female sexual anatomy.

CHAPTER 2
"OLD" MENOPAUSE & BEYOND

The second milestone in a women's life simply announces the end of reproductive capability. How did it become the millstone of physical disintegration or the death of sex?

2.1 ILL-OMENS & GHOST IMAGES

In a world where procreation is the primary feminine purpose, the post-menopausal woman is theoretically useless, and socially without function. Menopause was often identified with madness, making it ominous indeed: "... the end of the possibility of procreation could drive a menopausal woman mad, as she faced the loss of what was in reality her true female function."[14] No babies, no worth!

In a world reality where most people were dead by the time they were 40 or thereabouts, there was conceivably not that much time between menopause and death. So menopause might well have been the harbinger of immediate old age, and death itself, to a lot of women. Or else, some people got old at menopause and stayed old for decades until they did die.

Nowadays, we can easily live as many years after menopause as before, with an extended middle age before old age extremis sets in. The option of a very long middle age is what makes this subject so important to us today. What are we going to do with these years, sister?

Unhappy menopause! By word of mouth – mother to daughter, woman to woman, menopause is reported with sighs and shrugs – as if life as we know it were ending. It shakes a women's confidence and optimism; whether we believe it an illness or not, whether it leads to mania, depression, or emotional and mental breakdown – or not.

"... the end of the possibility of procreation could drive a menopausal woman mad, as she faced the loss of what was in reality her true female function."

Our very understanding of menopause is entangled with the dominating social and medical theories regarding ageing, sexuality and beauty. What comes from biology, environment or culture? What is fact; what is fiction? The theories set the context and the assumptions by which we live. They are the common truth of any period, and generate the fulfilling prophecies, for those who "believe" it is so. What we believe, we quite literally embody!

The theories fluctuate radically over time and culture, and often conflict, as do the prevailing stereotypes of post-menopausal women, reinforcing the pervasive dichotomies.

Join me on a condensed and terrible history tour of the last five centuries. These are the ghost images that inhabit our subconscious minds – the old stereotypes.

These are our psychological role models for menopause – and beyond!

Join me on a condensed and terrible history tour of the last five centuries. These are the ghost images that inhabit our subconscious minds – the old stereotypes.

2.2 BLOODLETTINGS, DARK HUMOURS & WITCHES

Early European medicine was based on the theory of four humours, and bloodletting was the favoured medical remedy for many maladies. As a result, menstruation, albeit a "curse", was considered beneficial as it provided "a monthly purging of those evil humours which might otherwise induce double reprehensible behaviour on the part of the weaker, less rational sex. The relationship between menstruation and the production of the ovum remained undiscovered until the mid-nineteenth century".[15]

If menstruation was healthy, its end was gloomy; "the evil humours remained present in the body, capable of adding to that complex of female wickedness which could turn aging women into witches".[16] According to one 17th-century French physician: "When seed and menstrual blood are retained in women besides (beyond) the intent of nature, they putrefie and are corrupted, and attain a malignant and venomous quality".[17]

Quite simply, in the 16th and 17th centuries, this malignant and venomous perception turned poor post-menopausal women into witches. That was the dominating stereotype – the lead role. It's not for nothing that most of the witches killed in Europe's dreadful witch hunts were "older women" – although "bewitchingly" beautiful younger women were included in the carnage.

By definition, a witch was two things: satanic and sexual; witches were

---

Quite simply, in the 16th and 17th centuries, this malignant and venomous perception turned poor post-menopausal women into witches.

"individuals who bound themselves diabolically to the devil through an infernal sexual pact".[18] "All witchcraft comes from carnal lust, which in women is insatiable," pronounced the major 1458 witchcraft manual, Witches' Hammer.[19] A 1550 view describes witches as "mostly old women who can find no lovers", and "have recourse to the devil to satisfy their appetites."[20]

Lest any of us miss the point here, you and I would probably have been defined as witches if we had been alive then. Anything over 40 would have been considered old, and hot flushes confirmed our melancholic and unstable nature. Poor women, weird women, widows with wealth, widows without wealth, smart women, healers, and herbalists – witches all!

Women themselves were often the accusers. According to Lois Banner, "the two derogatory names most commonly used by women against women in the medieval period were whore and witch. All women could be whores; all women could be witches."[21] Even today, women speak ill of each other too often.

Witches also invoke the terrible (?) idea of older women enjoying sex with younger men, an image which was/is considered fundamentally perverse and repulsive. "The existence of the mysterious menstrual blood in their bodies ... provided old witches with the power to attract young men."[22]

The abhorrence of cross-age sex, of the older woman with the younger man, haunts this whole history. Lois Banner's rich and erudite book

---

Lest any of us miss the point here, you and I would probably have been defined as witches if we had been alive then.

In Full Flower was originally motivated by her personal experiences in a relationship with a younger man. Drawing on history, mythology, literature and popular culture, the book examines the social and sexual status of ageing women in general, and specifically its affect on relationships with younger men.

Alternate roles of the time were as nurses or governesses, asexual intermediaries acting as benign agents of romance and social intrigue. Or they were malevolent intermediaries, the sexual procurer or "old bawd". (Older women were the "madams" at brothels long before the male pimp arrived to take over the oldest business.)

Privileged aristocratic women, or particularly feisty women, sometimes managed to attain positions of influence, but it was rare and against the mainstream.

Not much to choose from here in the overriding stereotypes of this era. 'Witch' one would you have been?

Older women were the "madams" at brothels long before the male pimp arrived to take over the oldest business.

2.3 SUBMISSION & SUBLIMATION; WIFE & GRANDMOTHER

With the era of rationality and the rise of the middle classes in the 18th and 19th centuries, woman become idealized and spiritualized as mother, embodying virtue and instilling morality in husband and children. The domesticated, patriarchal family evolved as a haven of security. Official sexuality was safely contained within marriage, where women were dutifully submissive.

Indeed, they seemed to have lost all interest in sex. "Women were not expected to feel desire and certainly not to experience an orgasm," was the standard 19th-century view of women's sexuality, reports historian Carl Degler.[23] "Male doctors (in the 1800s) were so convinced that women had no sexual interest that when it manifested itself, drastic measures were taken to subdue it, including excision of the sexual organs."[24]

Menstruation, having lost its "purgative benefits", became "an unfortunate failure in the bodily processes designed to build up a foetus", according to physicians of the time. This view was no help to womankind in general – our biology was still inherently wanting, but at least menopause was no longer dangerous and witch-making. It was re-imagined as a sort of liberation, "a regrouping of body forces away from childbirth toward other kinds of maternal, generative ends".[25] Now menstruation was out, and menopause was in, sort of.

Old women's lives were re-scripted. She could be an old maid who

---

With the era of rationality and the rise of the middle classes in the 18th and 19th centuries, woman become idealized and spiritualized as mother, embodying virtue and instilling morality in husband and children.

was negatively stereotyped and isolated; her sexuality safely under society's control by reason of its non-existence. Or she was the ageing grandmother, who now emerged as a positive persona. "Her emphasis on spirituality offered a justification for celibacy, domesticity or social involvement."[26] She was either doting on her grandchildren, engrossed in handiwork (embroidery was really big), home-making, or socially active, in support of the establishment – or social reform.

"Aging as an ethical experience which could enrich women and through this authorization render them beautiful was a common motif in nineteenth-century writings."[27] But sweet granny – like all little old ladies – was overtly asexual.

Female sexuality was hugely constrained and sublimated during this period, so dominated by Puritan and Victorian values. Women were no longer considered sexually voracious; if anything, many became invalids, and invalidism a lifestyle choice of the middle and upper classes.[28]

So here is the opening image for older women today – straight out of the 19th century. Righteous, moral, good granny – but not sexual in any way.

How many modern grannies are still living in that century – sexually speaking, that is? And as for the ageing spinster – enough said – no sex for her! Ageing women were not supposed to be sexual!

How many of us still resonate with that "truth" on some deep level? (Cross my heart. I promise I won't reveal your name if you tell me.)

Women were no longer considered sexually voracious; if anything, many became invalids, and invalidism a lifestyle choice of the middle and upper classes.

2.4 VITAL AGEING, REFORM & SARAH BERNHARDT

A temporary idealism reigned between 1890 and 1920, during a brief progressive period when the woman's rights movement was in full swing. It was buoyed by theories of vital ageing, positive attitudes towards menopause, and notions of women's superior morality extending from the 19th century.

There was also medical support for the view that there was no pathology associated with menopause, and that "most women experienced little discomfort".[29] Indeed, an 1893 medical observer recognized "that the absence of menstruation may be beneficial as an important aid to the preservation and increase of the vital forces".[30]

The US press talked about "the renaissance of the middle aged".[31] There was a "commitment to sweeping social change and positive response to the grandmother and the 'New Woman' as social types".[32]

Post-menopausal options were full of promise at the turn of the 20th century, prefiguring the rise of modern feminism that came later in the century – during our adulthood. Women were also entering and advancing in work, the professions, education, and the emergent reform movements. "In both numbers and energy, older women dominated women's Progressive reform organisations."[33] (Not much was said about their sexual life, though!)

Victorian attitudes to beauty and cosmetics relaxed. "Vogue magazine

---

Post-menopausal options were full of promise at the turn of the 20th century.

in the 1890s and 1900s published many articles about the new possibilities for ageing women and praised their new access to youthful standards of appearance."[34]

There were even celebrity role models for positive ageing, such as the famous Sarah Bernhardt, who was overtly sexual and luscious in her older years. "The 'over-ripe' sexual appearance of menopausal women was quite erotic and ... certain men – especially young men – could not resist them,"[35] wrote Enoch Kisch in his medical tome, The Sexual Life of Woman.

But the respite was brief indeed; old and new enemies threatened. Even our Mr Kisch unequivocally defined menopause as "that time in a woman's life at which her sexual activities come to their natural termination".[36] For him, procreation and sexuality for women were interchangeable phenomena.

Old notions of ageing women's dangerous deviant sexuality were revived, once again emphasizing the exclusively sexual nature of women. Now it could lead to lesbianism, nymphomania (a newly defined diagnosis of the 1920s), "unfortunate sexual experiences" – and younger men. "A real problem lay in the uncontrollable sexuality of older women and their desire for young men," wrote the reputable sexologist Havelock Ellis.[37]

Perhaps the increased social, economic, and educational mobility of women at the time generated competitive anxiety – anticipating the feminist movement to come. Already women's life options were

---

For him, procreation and sexuality for women were interchangeable phenomena.

being unlocked by fewer children, less death in childbirth, and the clustering of children in early years. There was time now for other things. "The Ladies' Home Journal noted old age disappearing as older women marched in parades, joined organisations, and founded literary clubs."[38]

The focus quickly shifted from vital ageing to a desperate holding on to youth at all costs. The subversive new enemy was the infatuation with youth. "In the 1920s sexuality became the desiderata of desirable self-construction and youth the preferred time of life. Advertising broadcast these messages worldwide."[39]

The nascent advertising industry produced images that captured the popular imagination – desirable erotic icons of youthful beauty and thin bodies. (In the 19th century plumpness had been the ideal look for married women, especially older women.)

The obsession with youthful beauty has had a huge and paralysing impact on the self-image of all women older than 30, but more so on post-menopausal women. Ironically, we who benefited most from the youth culture of the 1960s are being challenged to deal with its cruel impact – now, as we approach our 60s.

Our mirrors no longer reflect the ingénue of that time, nor the sophisticate of subsequent decades. Who is she in the mirror now – certainly not the fairest of them all, any more?

The focus quickly shifted from vital ageing to a desperate holding on to youth at all costs.

2.5 MEDICALIZED, PATHOLOGIZED & PSYCHOANALYSED

The menopause debate in the 20th century swung between menopause as pathology or as potential. Was it an illness, bringing inevitable breakdown of body and mind, or a time of renewed vigour, the "post-menopausal zest" so famously described and exemplified by anthropologist Margaret Mead?

Popular literature at the start of the century had portrayed a dangerous age for female protagonists between 40 and 50. They experienced mania, depression, and very odd behaviour, as if "slaves of an inevitable necessity".[40] This idea had a long, sad history, involving the believed connection between the uterus and the brain and "the tendency of aging women, with cold constitutions, to become melancholic".[41]

The list of common pathologies that filled mental institutions with post-menopausal patients is heart-rending: "involutional melancholia", "climacteric insanity", and "old maid's insanity".[42]

The other major pathology of menopause was sexuality itself, since by medical definition menopause was the "natural termination" of a woman's sex life. Remember Kisch? "Where the sexual impulse continues to manifest itself, it is pathological."[43] To be sexual after menopause was pathological – by medical definition.

"In the conflicting imagery of the first half of the 1900s, both the sexually deranged menopausal woman and her opposite,

---

The menopause debate in the 20th century swung between menopause as pathology or as potential.

the asexual menopausal women, could develop severe problems." Heightened sexuality could produce hysteria or nymphomania. But even women without (sexual) desire could fall into menopausal madness ... "a psychic sentimental state arising from a deep longing to be loved in the spiritual sense".[44] (See how longing is named lunacy!)

There is the basic physical fact; menstruation winds down and stops. There are some accompanying symptoms – for some. How widespread are these physical symptoms? How much are they just conditioned expectations now embodied in ailing flesh; how much is physiologically inherent in the human organism; how much is caused by physical neglect or negative cultural expectations?

Weight gain, for example, can have so many lifestyle causes. And yet we sigh "menopause", and eat the doughnuts. We fail to exercise, and generally abuse our poor bodies; we wouldn't do to our cars what we do to our bodies. The body may shift, but must it decline so?

Stuck with boring sex, unsatisfactory relationships, or disappointment with life generally, vaginas dry up.

Facing the midlife reality of a life not fully actualized, the bodies falter; facing a future without status, confidence wavers. Expecting decline, we decline.

A concurrent and contrary view was optimistic and forward-looking; "When the climacteric of middle life is reached, nature gives a fresh start and a fresh balance of power."[45] But this viewpoint got lost in history.

... But even women without (sexual) desire could fall into menopausal madness ...

Basically, the pathology version triumphed. The word menopause itself, derived from the Greek "meno meaning month and pausis, meaning ending",[46] was invented by French doctors. While neutral in itself – hey, it's better than "a dangerous age" – its official naming "plac[ed] the condition under medical management".[47]

Its various symptoms became the domain of medical specialists whose job it was to attend women through this period – once a year, please, at least – and, of course, through the post-menopause as well – until death do us part. The newly established field of gynaecology took control of menopause, as it had taken childbirth over from the midwives.

The growing size and structures of the medical profession in the early 20th century required an expanding patient population for economic viability. Menopausal and post-menopausal women formed the perfect client group – large numbers, ample finances, and vague symptoms. The medicalization of menopause was great for doctors.

Philip Wylie, a popular author of the time, painted a vicious misogynist view of this target market in 1942. "Never before has a great nation of brave and dreaming men absentmindedly created a huge class of idle, middle-aged women," which is accused of malingering (feigning illness in order to escape duty, work). "These caprices are ... menopausal at best; hot flashes, infantilism, weeping, sentimentality, peculiar appetite, and all the ragged reticule of tricks, wooings, wiles, subordined fornications."[48] It generated controversy, but his book had gone through 20 printings by 1955; people read it.

The newly established field of gynaecology took control of menopause, as it had taken childbirth over from the midwives.

Endocrinology, the new study of glands and hormones, joined gynaecology in describing an integrated, delicate feminine physiology that determined and dominated our character – and easily went awry. Hormone deficiencies and bone loss, and indeed just about every other ageing symptom, were added to the menopausal medical stew. (Oestrogen replacement therapy started in the 1940s.)[49]

The new psychology exacerbated an already bad situation. Freud's view of menopause "cemented the view that it was biological and pathological",[50] bringing much psychological insecurity. Who wouldn't become melancholic if they were sentenced to a lifetime of official, socially sanctioned meaninglessness?

"The negative views reached a nadir in the 1950s with the ubiquity of the Freudian interpretation ... by American psychoanalyst, Helene Deutsch",[51] which "identified a heightened sexuality as a major symptom of menopause".[52] She believed that menopause triggered a return to neurotic, adolescent behaviours.

In her view, "menopause was so difficult an experience that all menopausal women faced the possibility of developing sexual neuroses".[53] She "discounted the possibility that aging women, without the responsibilities of childrearing, might consider a lifestyle more devoted to self and society."[54] The only escape from the difficulties of menopause was "becoming doting, asexualized grandmothers".[55]

In 1949, even the brilliant Simone de Beauvoir was pessimistic, despite a classic French tradition of celebrating ageing women. She

---

The new psychology exacerbated an already bad situation. Freud's view of menopause "cemented the view that it was biological and pathological", bringing much psychological insecurity.

wrote that as women age and anticipate the end of beauty and love, "their minds became unbalanced" and "with bleak futures to anticipate, they turned into shrewish, paranoid versions of their former selves".[56]

Remnants of infantility join advanced senility to crowd out the middle range of mature womanhood, which thus becomes self-absorbed and stagnant, " observed the esteemed Erik Erikson in 1956 on the sad life cycle of many women.[57]

This is the miserable menopausal milieu into which we baby boomers were born. Our mothers and grandmothers were the sexually passive and dependent creatures of the 1950s. They anticipated, and for the most part lived through, this kind of menopause.

Although this might no longer be our conscious choice, the unexamined premises of these attitudes and beliefs have affected our menopause nonetheless. We have not so liberated ourselves as to be free of them – witness the explosion of symptoms and the dependence on medication.

When you visit your gynaecologist, or worse, the new endocrinologist and bone density specialist, do you come out feeling vaguely or overtly intimidated? Have you been solemnly presented with the expert outline of your inevitable deterioration, as they describe the sloping graph of increasing decay that ends in the grave?

Sexually speaking, these same medical experts are tentative and

---

We have not so liberated ourselves as to be free of them – witness the explosion of symptoms and the dependence on medication.

unconvincing, despite the now "politically correct" concession that moderate sex might be beneficial. It is better, at least, than the medical view of the 20th century that questioned whether the "congestive conditions" of the poor, sensitive, menopausal sexual organs were able to have sex at all that was not so "unbearable as to drive them to unfortunate sexual experiences".[58] That is, if they were not totally dried up!

Menopause is not an illness, and should not be solely or mainly a medical experience.

It is a life transition and an experience that is greater than a sum of shifting hormones and weakened bones. It is a deep, meaning-filled experience with potential for personal transformation. In short, it engenders soul. To truly believe that, and live that, we need a different attitude and mindset. We need to re-vision the vital ageing theory of the early 20th century – the one that lost the debate last time.

It is a life transition and an experience that is greater than a sum of shifting hormones and weakened bones. It is a deep, meaning-filled experience with potential for personal transformation.

2.6 ANOTHER KIND OF MENOPAUSE

The truth is we have no coherent image of a positive menopause. What would another kind of menopause look like?

We don't know how many of the problems associated with menopause are attributable to neglect of health in earlier life, and unresolved personal stuff to do with self, sexuality and ageing. We don't know how deeply the self-fulfilling prophecies of depressing cultural and medical expectations affect our bodies. How much is zeitgeist and how much the much maligned hormones alone? Is decline a given? Or is menopause an invitation to transformation?

In an obscure text of feminine Tantric Buddhism I found a tantalising reference to the practice of "deliberate and harmonious menopause".[59] This implies intent, anticipation and grace. What did these women know that we have lost so completely?

A deliberate and harmonious menopause!

The words intoxicate me. What secrets are they referring to that would make menopause "deliberate and harmonious" – truly a physical and spiritual gateway to the third phase of life? The translated verses are enigmatic; their meaning locked away in ambiguous poetic imagery.[60]

Another text describes menopause as the body's way of preparing for "worldly transcendence".[61]

The truth is we have no coherent image of a positive menopause. What would another kind of menopause look like?

These are profound concepts which go way beyond simply not viewing menopause as illness. They propose menopause as a positive experience of soul; an important life process in its own right, a graduation to something grand, and not simply a pathology to endure. Just as pregnancy and birth were meant to be.

Menopause is a transitional process, like adolescence; but adolescence is optimistic, and menopause rather grim. Major life-cycle transitions, like coming into life and leaving it, have been taken over by modern medicine. Instead of medicine just supporting these experiences, they have almost become the experience itself – one "smooth pharmaceutical flow" from birth control to post-menopause.[62]

What if we choose the mind/body perspective instead, and consider the very symptoms themselves as "body metaphors" calling us to reflect and review our lives, and not pathologies in need of obliteration?

If you blame it all on hormones and medically eliminate the symptoms, "you may miss the opportunity to know how you feel about yourself and your life", suggests Jean Shinoda Bolen.[63]

Restlessness and irritability may be a challenge to make inner and/or outer life changes – medication will calm us down, but what about the life change this restlessness signals? Hot flashes may signify rising kundalini energy, a surge of strength, a call to power and transformation – perhaps we should assimilate them, not squash them? Dry genitals challenge our relationship to love, sexuality, the person we are with, and the person we have become.

Menopause is a transitional process, like adolescence; but adolescence is optimistic, and menopause rather grim.

We have spent a lifetime unconsciously expecting this change; they told us so. Did we ever examine what we were expecting? Did we ever, before the event, review our core cultural beliefs about the meaning and nature of menopause?

The deliberate menopause of the immortal Tantric Buddhist sisters involved spiritual practices of some kind. And, as we will learn, meditation, spiritual practices, energy circulation ... are all essentially psychosomatic practices, affecting mind, soul – and body.

I have just "done" menopause. The only "symptom" I experienced was hot flashes, which I do not find at all problematic. I think of them as Lesley Kenton's power surges, or kundalini rushes, or at least as an inner cleansing, keeping my skin moist and supple. Would that I had known the secrets of a "deliberate and harmonious" menopause!

How different will it be for a new generation of women, living their adult life expecting a "deliberate and harmonious" menopause?

How would that self-fulfilling prophecy play out in the real lives of real women? What would be the metaphoric and psychological characteristics of a "deliberate and harmonious menopause" – and what the physical manifestations?

I look forward to another generation of women to elucidate this alternative. All I can teach is what menopause is NOT. It is not a medical experience, nor an omen of decrepitude, madness, or uselessness. All I know is that it IS a process of soul.

Did we ever, before the event, review our core cultural beliefs about the meaning and nature of menopause?

Ideally, the transition of menopause should be completed by a joyous, confident entry into the next phase of life, the third face of the Goddess. This would involve self-reflection that redefined self, life, spirit, and sex. And there lies the rub – or rather the chafe!

It is alarming how so many currently menopausal and post-menopausal women are suffering from dried-up vaginas, politely called vaginal atrophy, on the one hand – and urinary incontinence on the other. We are told that this is "normal" to menopause – to be expected, inevitable – like destiny!

These vaginal and pelvic symptoms are so pervasive, it makes me think that we are really suffering from a profound historical devaluation of our sexual parts which is aeons old; the belief in an inferior biology that has now become poetically embodied in our poor "fleeced and drybaked cunt".[64]

Come, let us go down there and examine these nether parts – the parts we think we know – and the parts we don't!

How different will it be for a new generation of women, living their adult life expecting a "deliberate and harmonious" menopause?

CHAPTER 3
SEXUAL ANATOMY AS DESTINY

The world view of more than two millennia is that female anatomy is inferior to the more "perfect" male anatomy; and is the negative of the male, not itself an entity; yet, "delicate and capricious", it rules our functioning. We "were not made in the image of God" [65] *according to Augustine and theologians even wondered whether we had a soul at all.*

To this destiny we have been held hostage. Are we going to continue to accept on some deep level that our biology is inferior?

3.1 A DESTINY OF INFERIOR ORGANS

"Just as mankind is the most perfect of all animals, so within mankind the man is more perfect than the woman ... The woman is less perfect than the man in respect to the generative parts ... Indeed, you ought not to think that our Creator would purposely make half the whole race imperfect and, as it were, mutilated, unless there was to be some great advantage in such mutilation." [66]

So said Galen, authoritative Greek-born physician of the second century AD, whose teachings dominated ancient medicine. Is it so different today? Does this idea not linger and lurk in our modern mindset?

Two thousand years later Freud still imagined women as castrated males, and considered our clitoris an atrophied penis. We are driven, supposedly, by penis envy and a castration complex, terms which have become part of popular psycho-speak. Without denigrating the enormous value of Freud's total body of psychological work, his penis envy and castration stuff miss the point.

It was not the discovery that I might be castrated or that I might "envy" the male for his penis that disturbed, but the uncomfortable a priori knowing, long before little me ever set eyes on a penis, that my genitals were inherently, essentially not good enough. (The closest I came to penis envy was seeing my little boy gleefully urinate in all directions when outdoors or in a parking lot, and my little girl having to crouch coyly to do her thing.)

Two thousand years later Freud still imagined women as castrated males, and considered our clitoris an atrophied penis.

We imbibe this age-old view of feminine genitals as something ugly and inherently inferior. It haunts us, as if our mothers, and the mothers of our mothers down history, had passed on this ancient shame and disgust – a subtle transmission of thought, of knowing, with a look, a sigh, a hesitant hand.

Freud considered shame a "feminine characteristic par excellence [that] has as its purpose, we believe, the concealment of genital deficiency".[67]

The dishonour of the ages – inherently inferior genitals (Nancy Friday recalls that her vagina was named the Cloaca, which is Latin for sewer) [68] – casts a long, punishing shadow. It is no wonder, then, that we are not at peace with our genitals; so many negative thoughts, images, and beliefs revolve around this area, aversions and revulsions which impact our self-image, our sex life, and our psyche.

We are deeply disconnected from our genitals. We have almost numbed them out. If you fully love, and accept, and are comfortable with your genitals, without the faintest unease at all – then perhaps you skip the rest of this section. (Personally, I would love to know how many women like that there are.)

If our deepest inner confusion starts with our sexual parts, just how far can our heads, hearts, and instincts actually take us? Fear of sex, said Nancy Friday, is what modern feminism did not address.[69] So let's re-examine that place which first and forever after defined us as female. Let's look at our genitals.

If our deepest inner confusion starts with our sexual parts, just how far can our heads, hearts, and instincts actually take us?

At least as we get to the other side of 50/60/70, we should take another (final?) look. There is no way we can be sexual forever without a more positive attitude to ageing, our bodies – and our sexual parts.

They looked, they saw, and they said (without too much disappointment, we hope), "It's a girl!" What did they see?

Did they see a sewer, did they see something ugly, or something missing, or did they see something lovely? In some ancient texts female genitals were called "os sacrum" – the sacred mouth. Where did sacred become Sewer? (When my first child was born, I received a little cactus plant from a family member, saying in congratulations, "a little prick first time". As if it mattered! And it sort of did.)

Camille Paglia describes our secret places thus: "In aesthetic terms, female genitals are lurid in colour, vagrant in contour and architecturally incoherent. Male genitals, on the other hand, though they risk ludicrousness by their rubbery indecisiveness, have a rational mathematical design, a syntax."[70]

At least there is a measure of equivalence between "incoherent" and "indecisive", although men do have a very immediate relationship with theirs; handling their (rational) piece daily and seeing it directly. They size up each others' pieces in the locker room. We can't see ours – or each others' – directly, and our daily touching is quite superficial.

How are we supposed to love this most intimate, wondrous thing that "they" call the sewer?

In some ancient texts female genitals were called "os sacrum" – the sacred mouth.

3.2 LOVE MY YONI, LOVE MYSELF

Down there, my private parts, the slit, the gash, the cleft, the wound, the sewer, our own mothers' (and mothers' mothers' mothers', no doubt) distaste and shame around it. "Man's great misfortune was to have been born from woman's stinking private parts," proclaimed a prince-bishop of the Inquisition,[71] reflecting and reinforcing a deep cultural distaste. What chance did we have here?

I dislike all the words used, including vulva, great cleft, pussy, pudenda, and cunt. Vagina is barely OK, I suppose, but technically it refers to the sheath inside only. The place between our legs is unseen, unmanageable, and deeply suspect. The idea lingers that it is somewhat dirty, offensive, less than.

What other awful names are there? And let's not even contemplate the consequences of such awful attitudes, which lead to genital mutilation in women in some parts of the world. Even now, all the words make me uncomfortable, as if centuries of disgust and scorn still echo in every one of them. How were we ever going to feel the grace of feminine essence, without a worthwhile name?

One of the biggest breakthroughs for me was doing an exercise to look at my own sexual organs with a hand mirror. Does the thought disgust us? Well, it shouldn't. Why shouldn't we know how we look "down there"? It's an exercise worth doing.

The various folds, the opening, the contours, the colours! This is me,

---

Down there, my private parts, the slit, the gash, the cleft, the wound, the sewer, our own mothers' (and mothers' mothers' mothers', no doubt) distaste and shame around it.

this is you! Even then I worried that somehow the lack of regularity of the various folds (my "vagrant contours") might mean there was something wrong with me.

At that time I came upon the most fabulous book called The Yoni, by Rufus Camphausen.[72] Yoni is the Sanskrit word for female genitalia, which is so far superior to any of the ugly words we Westerners use to describe this unnamed, not named, badly named section of a girl's anatomy.

The word is on a respectful par with the word 'Lingam' for penis, and both were objects of symbolic worship and reverence in the best of the ancient East. That's right. Way back, in the East (and in the West, also, in pre-patriarchal times), the Yoni was worshipped as the sacred symbol of the great goddess. How can we then feel badly about something of such reverence? But we do, because we have forgotten it is something sacred. Little cat indeed!

Camphausen's book is a work of art, and includes exquisite photographs of some real-life Yonis. It made me want to laugh out loud in gleeful delight. Suddenly my private parts had a context. We get to accept the look of our faces one way or the other, because we see other faces all the time. But we don't ever get the chance to see each others' "private parts". They have been a dark continent for all but midwives and doctors.

These Yonis were all so beautiful in their way that it made me feel

---

Way back, in the East (and in the West, also, in pre-patriarchal times), the Yoni was worshipped as the sacred symbol of the great goddess.

instantly reconciled to mine. Utter relief, really.

Yes, I was willing to love my Yoni, love myself. So we are now, theoretically at least, getting reconciled to our divine Yonis. Right!

A teacher [73] with great knowledge in these matters pointed out to me that when we import a foreign word for something that has complex emotional loadings, we take the lyrical foreign tone to imply a squeaky-clean, dirt-free meaning on its home turf. And this is probably not true. He suggests that it's exactly the word "cunt" that we should embrace.

Germaine Greer would agree with him. Decades ago she wrote, " It is time to dig CUNT and women must dig it first."[74]

They might be right. But for now, for myself, I'll hold onto my Yoni!

Yes, I was willing to love my yoni, love myself.

3.3 EVE'S SECRETS & VAGINA 101

We still contend psychologically with the heritage of the questionable biology of the past. The accepted theory of female anatomy had not changed in more than 20 centuries until Josephine Lowndes Sevely published her ground-breaking book Eve's Secret in 1987, that did not take the world by storm, but should have.

Lowndes Sevely [75] asserts that we haven't even got the anatomy right, as the theory of female sexual anatomy "did not develop as part of the normal scientific process". Instead, "it was based on preconceptions about the sexes that went back to the ancient Greeks' and early Judaic/Christian writers' notions of sexual inequality and of woman as an incomplete version of man".

She traces these ideas in philosophy and religion and in early Western medical texts. The physician who first described the female genitals – who were, of course, all men – did so from the same male point of view, as an inferior version of the male's.

The clitoris was described for the first time only in 1561, by Renaissance scientist Fallopio (of Fallopian tubes fame), who wrote: "Truly, our anatomists completely neglected it and do not even speak of it. This small part corresponds to the male penis ... This very private part, small in size and hidden in the very fatty part of the pubis, has remained unknown to the anatomists, so that up to now from the preceding years I am the first to describe it, ... there is not a good knowledge about it." [76]

We still contend psychologically with the heritage of the questionable biology of the past.

To clarify a vast confusion, Lowndes Sevely conducted detailed research of both male and female genitalia, including a study of the female urethra and vagina. Here is Vagina 101 – a new look at our private parts (sic!) a la Lowndes. She established:

- The clitoral tip has its true counterpart in a male clitoris inside the penis, both of which she named the Lowndes crowns: "The male structure is the part that fills with blood and brings about erection, a capsule-like part called the corpora cavernosa, meaning literally 'cavernous bodies'."[77]

- The clitoris should be seen as the small visible part of a complex vaginal structure, as it is connected to deep, hidden structures under the skin that substantially reflect the interior structures of the penis.

- The counterpart to the penile glans is the soft, relatively prominent but until now unnamed area from the clitoris and around and between the urethra opening and the carina (the edge of the glans) which defines the beginning of the vagina, both extremely sensitive to touch.

- The differences in organisational structure reflect a male fusion/female diffusion, which parallels yin/yang symmetry rather than a superior/inferior hierarchy... (the man as "more perfect than the woman").

- She emphasizes the existence of female prostate glands (popularized as the G-spot) and female ejaculation (widely accepted in earlier times, but denied in more recent ones), and its challenging

---

The differences in organisational structure reflect a male fusion/female diffusion, which parallels yin/yang symmetry rather than a superior/inferior hierarchy ...

implication that the female urethra, like the male one, is also a sexual organ. "Are female sexual fluids released through the urethra?" she asks, and answers affirmatively.

- She proposes that the female sexual response is complex and involves the clitoris, the urethra, and the vagina functioning as a unit, which she named the C.U.V response.

- The vagina should be seen as an entity of interrelated parts. "Once the vagina is perceived as an entity of sexual parts, in the way that the penis has always been perceived, it becomes clear that the true counterparts are not the penis and clitoris ... the true counterparts are the penis and the vagina."[78] (No atrophied penis, please, Dr Freud.)

- She compares a man's erection in readiness for orgasm to the C.U.V. response in women, ie the simultaneous response of the clitoris, the urethra, the vagina, and their related structures. "When the C.U.V. response has been elicited, a woman experiences heightened sensitivity. At this stage, the C.U.V. structures become a unified sensory organ, through which a woman perceives sensations of touch and pressure"[79] – a female organ of unified parts.

So! We now have a divine Yoni and a respectably equivalent biology.

Are we getting more comfortable with our "private parts" here? Can we touch ourselves with greater tenderness, and respect, and wonder?

So! We now have a divine Yoni and a respectably equivalent biology.

3.4 NO LONGER PASSIVE PLUMBING

The profound Julius Evola, in his book on the metaphysics of sex, makes a remarkable statement: "In fact, we believe that during the course of history a physiological atrophy has occurred in feminine sexuality."[80]

He is not talking about dry menopausal vaginas, but a general atrophy throughout adult life of the vaginal muscles themselves. Generations of women with weak sex muscles who simply didn't know how to use them properly – or feel them at all!

He describes an ancient "active participation of woman in coitus", that is now "unusual in European women".[81] He says that Oriental women "are closest to the ancient type in their physiological behaviour"[82] – or highly sexed (Western) women (the bad ones, remember?). Somehow our sexual plumbing became passive.

Active participation means "rhythmic contractions of the vagina and uterus, like an aspiration or suction, and of spasmodic automatic movements with their own special wavelike contractions based on particular slow rhythmic tonic waves".[83] Simply put, it means controlling our constrictor cunni – the muscle that constricts the vagina; activating our plumbing by pulling in, up and out! Not our stomach, but our pelvic floor! So utterly basic and straightforward.

This training was part of the erotic teaching in the East; no such training in the West. Passive sexuality has also meant flaccid, un-

---

The profound Julius Evola, in his book on the metaphysics of sex, makes a remarkable statement: "In fact, we believe that during the course of history a physiological atrophy has occurred in feminine sexuality."

used vaginal muscles. Do we know how to use our muscles down there? Is it any wonder that we have an epidemic of prolapsed uteruses and urinary incontinence – whether we have had children or not? (Perhaps menopausal atrophy is in part a consequence of this lifetime of non-use, or, at the very least, incorrect use.)

Dr Andrew Kegel developed his Kegel pelvic floor exercises in the 1940s as a self-help alternative to surgery. Simple exercises of vaginal squeezing and relaxing increase awareness of the vaginal muscles, as well as tone and strengthen them. They are very similar to the exercises of the ancient erotic traditions.

They enhance our sexuality, increase our pleasure, stop incontinence, and prevent pelvic organ prolapse – all of which have become common "symptoms" of menopause and ageing. Yet all we need is consistently to exercise "down there" – and use it when we make love.

Isn't it extraordinary how, by making our "private parts" into the sewer, we have numbed our minds to down under, and, at the same time, virtually atrophied our musculature. Our vaginas are active, amorous spaces, which need to be activated by – not the handsome prince, not the saviour, not the doctor – but ourselves.

So pull up, ladies! These exercises can be facilitated with devices such as an egg-shaped object (used in the East), or more sophisticated vaginal weights, some developed by gynaecologists, which can be bought. Passive plumbing indeed!

Isn't it extraordinary how, by making our "private parts" into the sewer, we have numbed our minds to down under, and, at the same time, virtually atrophied our musculature.

3.5 OUR "HYSTERICAL" TRAVELLING UTERUS

Another anatomical "reality" that has persisted in Western medical lore since ancient Greece was that the female uterus becomes displeased and displaced, and wanders through the body, negatively influencing the brain (I kid you not!). "Hysteria" is derived from the Greek word for uterus.

In a fit of "womb furie",[84] the female uterus went travelling through the body, causing all manner of emotional disturbances – hence hysteria, hysterical – and hysterectomy.

The mental condition of hysteria afflicted legions of women of all ages throughout the patriarchal centuries, and was considered the most common disease after fever. In menopause, specifically, "the belief was that the failure to menstruate caused the uterus to travel around the body, eventually negatively influencing the brain".[85]

The descriptions of hysterical patients paint a caricature of the feminine. Old treatments included bed rest, binding, beating, purging, bloodletting, and, in worse cases, hysterectomy and/or clitoridectomy.

A kinder treatment evolved in the 19th century, when hysteria became a veritable epidemic, especially in the white middle classes. The doctor massaged the genitals until there was a healing convulsion and moist spasms (an orgasm by any other name), which relieved the patient for a while – until the next appointment. Hysteria was considered chronic and incurable, requiring ongoing treatment.

Another anatomical "reality" that has persisted in Western medical lore since ancient Greece was that the female uterus becomes displeased and displaced, and wanders through the body, negatively influencing the brain.

Electric vibrators were developed in the mid 19th century to help the overworked doctors and ease the hysterical women. They were even marketed to women at home for self-treatment, and were advertized in consumer catalogues and magazines. (There were vibrators in the house before vacuum cleaners.) However, by 1930 vibrators had gone underground, and were not openly advertized again until they re-emerged as sex toys in the 1960s.

The treatment of hysteria was taken over by psychology, and Freud pretty much evolved his world-shattering theories based on his work with hysterical (and frigid) women. And, well, we should be grateful for that.

He explained hysteria as the physical and psychological expression of inner psychic conflicts about sexuality. (Psyche turned into soma.) He explored his patients' personal history for clues, practised the talking cure (hugely innovative for its time), and developed psychoanalysis.

In my view, these legions of hysterical women were literally quivering with centuries of misogynist repressions, bursting to break out of the traumatized collective psyche; an epidemic erupting out of the universal unconscious where the goddess of myth lay buried.

In the good doctor's own words, "The character of hysterics shows a degree of sexual repression in excess of the normal quantity, an intensification of resistance against the sexual instinct (which we have already met with in the form of shame, disgust and morality), and

---

The treatment of hysteria was taken over by psychology, and Freud pretty much evolved his world-shattering theories based on his work with hysterical (and frigid) women.

what seems like an instinctive aversion on their part to any intellectual consideration of sexual problems.

"This trait ... is not uncommonly screened by the existence of a second constitutional character present in hysteria, namely the predominant development of the sexual instinct. Psychoanalysis ... reveals the pair of opposites by which it is characterised – exaggerated sexual craving and excessive aversion to sexuality."[86] She wanted and she didn't want: another version of the old dichotomy!

Modern psychology succeeded in shifting hysteria from the realm of superstition. You could say it cured the mass hysteria; by 1952, it was officially declared a non-disease.

Freud introduced the concept of libido, the psychic energy expressed through sexuality that lies at the root of every living individual, and drives our desires and impulses. It can be repressed, expressed, controlled, or transmuted. But it exists – a priori!

Psychology helped to make conscious the compulsion of instincts hidden in the unconscious psyche. Basically ordinary people could now understand their behaviours and symptoms as expressions of underlying psychic/psychological conflict. Jung introduced the idea of the collective unconscious, which illuminated the universality of dream images and personal unconscious content.

The hysteric's subjugated sexuality was now the very stuff of the modern age, just waiting for the 1960s to burst out on to the world

---

The hysteric's subjugated sexuality was now the very stuff of the modern age, just waiting for the 1960s to burst out on to the world stage of the post-war baby boomers.

stage of the post-war baby boomers. The sexual liberation of that period was a huge and abrupt cultural change. Perhaps we forget now just how radical and fundamental it was - this sexual break from the past.

However, before we get too satisfied with this development, we need to ask ourselves why, with hysteria safely unplugged, we now have a virtual epidemic of hysterectomies, now the second most frequent surgery among American women, with caesarean section delivery being first. One in three women in the United States has had a hysterectomy by age 60!

If our hysterical uteruses are no longer travelling through our bodies affecting our brains, why are so many women having them cut out?

So much for the destiny of our anatomy, and the inevitable functional consequences of an unambiguous, clearly (mis)understood, scientifically definitive physiology. Is it any wonder there is confusion?

If our hysterical uteruses are no longer travelling through our bodies affecting our brains, why are so many women having them cut out?

3.6 ORGASM & EJACULATION

We cannot end this "anatomy as destiny" section without a discussion of orgasm and ejaculation. There has been no definitive biology on these matters either – and much misinformation.

We grew up in the period when women had only just begun to exit their sexual closets. But even the most radical sexual revolutionary was brought up by parents under the influence of 19th century norms, by which being feminine meant the absence of sexual desire. (If they "enjoyed" sex, they were very, very bad!)

In our post-war cradles we still imbibed large doses of these terrible taboos, which probably affect us more in our "old age" than in our revolutionary youth. Like Nancy Friday's idea about healing the inner good mother/bad mother split, it needs addressing now.

Much happened in the 20th century Western world in terms of sexual theory.

It was only in the 1940s that Dr Alfred Kinsey began investigating and statistically recording real sexual behaviour. His Sexual Behaviour in the Human Female, first published in 1953, reflected a wide range of such behaviour.

His subjects were born during a period from before 1900 to 1929 – when the male-on-top missionary position was traditional in European and American cultures, and was considered "the only biologically

---

Much happened in the 20th century Western world in terms of sexual theory.

normal position",[87] the reverse being evidence of personality disorder. Of those born between 1920 and 1929, 52% had had some sex with the woman on top, compared to 35% of those born before 1900.

It was only from 1957 through to 1965 that Masters and Johnson first directly observed sex in a laboratory and reported their findings. (They were also the first to research the sexuality of "older adults", concluding that with good health, good sex has no end. This finding had little general impact though.)

There was a lot of ponderous professional deliberation among medical doctors and psychologists about the nature of female orgasm. They seriously analysed differences between a clitoral and vaginal orgasm, which were seen as separate and distinct responses rather than biologically linked, a la Eve's Secret. Was the clitoris the main focal point of female sexual sensitivity – or not?

It was only in the early 1980s that the work of John Perry and Beverly Whipple regarding the G-spot and female ejaculation was published and popularized.

Basically, there is an extremely sensitive spot inside the vagina (named the G spot after the first doctor to describe it), which can be stimulated to orgasm and which can lead to a liquid ejaculation through the urethra that is not urine. The urethral glands function as a female prostate, and the ejaculate is chemically similar to male ejaculate, sans the sperm. Eve's Secret was published in 1987.

It was only from 1957 through to 1965 that Masters and Johnson first directly observed sex in a laboratory and reported their findings.

Older writers and folklore alluded to these secret waters. But the notion of female ejaculation was lost over the centuries, to the point where it was deemed physiologically impossible, or a symptom of a pathological disorder often confused with urinary incontinence – and valid grounds for divorce. (Pornographic use of urinating is a debased form of this very great secret.)

Even today, unless people, including doctors themselves, have had direct experience of female ejaculation, many continue to deny its existence. Some women may have an aversion because it initially feels like you want to pee. It also requires a great degree of physical and emotional surrender, of comfort with your body, your sex, your life, your partner. It is, however, real – and very nice indeed!

Apparently there is also a U-spot (sensitive tissue on either side of the urethral opening), and an A-Spot (just above the cervix, deep inside), discovered in the 1990s.[88]

And there are still 23 other letters left in the alphabet.

But let's get back to orgasm, for now.

While all these medical sex mavens of the 20th century were busy with their investigations, definitions and debates, how did our orgasms evolve from the '60s, or whenever we began, until now? Did they change, evolve, grow? Did they deepen? Were they explosive or gentle, great jerky contractions or a "sweet yielding softness",[89] vibrations, surges, waves of sensation?

Even today, unless people, including doctors themselves, have had direct experience of female ejaculation, many continue to deny its existence.

Did these medical debates, in as much as bits and bytes were reported in the media, affect us? The debates on orgasm were generally very genitally directed, leading to various distinctions between muscular spasms localized in the genitals and contractions in the body. The former were sometimes called orgasm, and the latter climax, but they were also used interchangeably.

Generally, Western sex was pointedly goal-directed to the man's ejaculation, which was usually identified with orgasm. Genital focus was the only focus. Her "pleasure", if at all, was usually by virtue of his patience, his skill, his actions, something he was supposed to give her – but it, too, became goal obsessed. An unfair burden on both; sometimes she wasn't sure if what she felt was an orgasm or not – hence the faking.

Although Kinsey had observed the distinction between male orgasm and ejaculation,[90] the proposition of orgasm as an erotic sensation not necessarily linked with the overt release of sexual fluids, of the two as physiologically distinct processes, was quite radical for Westerners.

(There had been 19th century European proponents of an extended and ecstatic love-making technique called Karezza, but it did not become mainstream.) Besides offering great opportunities to deepen and lengthen love-making, this phenomenon held much deeper repercussions. Once we are not focused on liquid emissions, the metaphysical dimensions of a full-body experience present itself.

Generally, Western sex was pointedly goal-directed to the man's ejaculation, which was usually identified with orgasm. Genital focus was the only focus.

This introduces language of a different order and higher frequency: vibrations, pulses, streams of sensation, waves, energy release, energy exchanges, and energy permeation. This language begins to resemble that of the ancient esoteric traditions of Tantra and Yoga (India), and Taoism (China), which spoke of this energy stuff a long time ago.

It was only in the 1960s that these ancient Eastern sexual practices were introduced to the West. Accessible books and teachers did not reach the general public until late in the 1980s, and the 1990s.

The information remains insufficiently assimilated and distilled into our understanding, our culture, and our real lives to make a meaningful difference, notwithstanding that bookshelves and magazines are full of "10 Easy Steps to Ecstasy" and "Tantra in Ten Minutes", and the like. A typically superficial fast-food approach to what is a discipline and a life path!

The best that the West provided in this respect was poor William Reich in the early 20th century. A student of Freud, he explored ideas about a sexual and energy economy. We become ill and psychologically troubled when our (sexual) energy gets bound up in chronic muscular tension – in our neuroses – preventing full surrender to the orgasmic reflex which was the goal of Reichian therapy.

Respiratory waves produced an undulating movement of the body that Reich called the orgasm reflex. Emotional health was the capacity for full surrender to these spontaneous and involuntary movements

---

It was only in the 1960s that these ancient Eastern sexual practices were introduced to the West.

in the sexual act.⁹¹ Reich got a bit lost when he tried to literally collect and store this "orgone" energy in a box; he died early. I wonder what he would have done with Taoist and Tantric knowledge. I feel kind of sorry for him; he was so close, in a way – but so far off, as well.

The Tantra and Taoist traditions offer us the deep and incontrovertible insight that sex extends beyond the genitals and ejaculatory fluids, and involves flows and streams of energy that are psychosomatic in nature; sexuality as a spiritual activity. We can learn much from their teachings. But the story doesn't end here.

While the Tantra and Taoist methods are profound, they are steeped in the images, rituals, and religious symbols of their culture, exotic metaphors which do not easily resonate for us. Nor should they; they carry their own cultural baggage. We need to find our own living metaphors to apply and integrate these sexual wisdoms in another way.

All of this new information, the developments of modern Western sexology and the ancient Eastern sexual secrets, only became available to us through our own adulthood – when we were also very busy with career and family and responsibilities. Historically speaking, it is all still relatively new. And then we hit menopause!

Yet here lies the path that can redeem and complete the genuine gifts of the 1960s – the sexual liberation of our youth. What else did we learn about sex during the decades of our adulthood? How sexually

---

We need to find our own living metaphors to apply and integrate these sexual wisdoms in another way.

mature and enlightened do we think we are?

Remember how it was way back then, when we were young, most of us, the teenage daughters of the 1960s, affected one way or the other by the Age of Aquarius and popular new notions of sexual freedom? Whether we were at Woodstock or not; whether we pretended or not!

We were going to be different to our mothers. We were OK with sex; we were going to be cool, modern, weren't we? Now that we are older, and have been sexually active for decades, we think we know sex. No longer naïve, are we now jaded, worn out, cynical – or passionate and still in love with love? Promiscuity in itself does not make for sexual skill; nor does marital sex ensure style.

Perhaps the hard truth is that the revolution of the 1960s failed to fulfil its promise because it was an inverted version of a masculine prototype – assertive, goal oriented, manipulative. It might have been free, but where was the soul, and where a feminine focus? What would a liberated feminine sexuality be like?

Come let us review **SEX** – what we think we know about sex, its nature, drives, explanations, and motivations, and examine other uses and purposes of sex, in cultures other than our own.

Perhaps the hard truth is that the revolution of the 1960s failed to fulfil its promise because it was an inverted version of a masculine prototype – assertive, goal oriented, manipulative.

CHAPTER 4
SEX: SACRED & PROFANE

*Sex covers ALL aspects of being human – and
more; it is physical and it is metaphysical.
"The metaphysics of sex survives in the very
cases where, in looking at wretched mankind
and the vulgarity of infinite lovers of infinite races –
endless masks and individuations of the Absolute Man
seeking the Absolute Woman in a turn of the circle
of animal generation – it is hard to overcome
a feeling of disgust and revolt and the temptation
to accept the biological and physical theory which
says that human sexuality springs from the life of
instincts and mere animality."* [92]

4.1 HUMAN SEX IS ...

- **Sex is physical** ... Definitely! It is biological, and relates to body instinct and body awareness. We use our bodies, we touch our bodies. No real problem here. Sex is overtly physical.

- **Sex is emotional** ... Well, yes, it's about feeling and emotion, when it is a common experience of two people in love – or hate, or power, lust, control, or fear, or submission. We feel excited, stimulated, happy, distressed. No real problem here. Sex is also emotional.

- **Sex is mental** ... Tricky! We tend to not think of sex as something mental, cerebral, or intellectual, especially, when it is so overtly ... well, physical and instinctive.

But think about this. It is our thoughts and attitudes and beliefs about sex that deeply affect us. These are mental processes. All our repressed attitudes, beliefs, inhibitions, compulsions, and self-loathing around sexuality get activated in our sexuality unless we have cleared them. Yea, this is mental, mind, brain, body-mind stuff – the province of psychology.

If we were more conscious about the mental aspects of sex, we could put our minds to good 'sexual' use in many ways.

One way is psychological, consciously working to clear our subconscious complexes and issues about sex.

All our repressed attitudes, beliefs, inhibitions, compulsions, and self-loathing around sexuality get activated in our sexuality unless we have cleared them.

Another is purely practical and functional, we could study the "arts of erotic love", long known in the East, with discrimination, discernment, and creativity.

The last way relates to thoughtful and intelligent relationship, behaving with respect and consideration to our sexual partner. This is no longer a bang-bang situation. Indeed, when a man's (or woman's) brains (or thinking processes) operate from their genitalia alone, everything does becomes base. The genitals are a given but what about a sensuous mind – or a sexual heart?

Yes, sex is also mental. Think about that!

- **Sex is spiritual** ... So is sex also spiritual? No, no, no, exclaims our cultural conditioning! This is the really difficult one for most people to relate to sexuality; especially when the physical (soma) is defined by the absence of spirit.

The best way our culture has dealt with this is to sanction and sanctify sex within marriage alone – and thereby control the whole thing. If one gets married within a religious context, the energy of the sacred is introduced, and perhaps the early sex rides on that wave of blessing, prayer, and ritual. But is it sustainable, if the fundamental beliefs, deep in our core DNA, decree that sexuality, physicality, is inherently sinful, wrong, dirty, bad – as intrinsically non-spiritual? If we still believe on any level that Eve sinned!

The joining together of bodies perceived as evil flesh. and that of bodies perceived as temples of the soul, are profoundly different unions.

The joining together of bodies perceived as evil flesh. and that of bodies perceived as temples of the soul, are profoundly different unions. Tantric lovemaking describes man worshipping woman as deity, her sexual organ as throne of enlightenment, and her sexual fluid as divine nectar. That is beautiful.

If we are physical, emotional, mental, and spiritual beings, should not sex then dance in all these dimensions – brain and genitals, heart and substance, sensual sensations, amorous excitations – and ecstatic devotion?

Has your sexuality over the years operated from all these levels? Which has been the primary aspect? Which the least?

What if the very energy of sex is itself divine? This is a big one, but it is at the core of everything. Certainly this is my premise. Sexuality is sacred. Sex is a spiritual activity.

What would that actually mean in our real lives, as post-menopausal women in the 21st century, whether we are married or not, in a relationship or not, religious or not?

... should not sex then dance in all these dimensions – brain and genitals, heart and substance, sensual sensations, amorous excitations – and ecstatic devotion?

4.2 THE BASICS
(INCLUDING THE BAD, SAD & DUTIFUL)

What are the basic purposes of sex in human society, and how do they fit in with being post-menopausal? Is its essential nature and purpose rooted in biology, psychology, sociology, anthropology, religion? There are many viewing points; and each becomes the symbolic lens through which we will perceive and experience our sexuality.

- **Viewing Point 1:** Sex is purely about procreation, a "biological end purpose",[93] an instinct of the species to reproduce; women are mere "bait for procreation".[94]

This view holds that sex is a natural, primitive instinct, the simple biological mechanism of the species. This sex would require a localized bang-bang act at the right time (like animals on heat), without the kissing and rapturous merging of breath and bodies, and would cease altogether once procreation is complete.

We have to get over the sex-for-procreation thing as primary. If procreation and reproduction are the main purposes of sex, and the only female function, then once we have done menopause, lady, it is over!

It is a short leap of logic to the widely held conclusion that, having lost her true female function, post-menopausal woman might be "driven mad by the end of the possibility of procreation".

If procreation and reproduction are the main purposes of sex, and the only female function, then once we have done menopause, lady, it is over!

By this definition, menopausal women are finished – no longer truly female, with no biological purpose, and an out-of-whack, utterly useless sexual hormonology making them crazy. Any sexual interest is deeply problematic. This is what the old medical and cultural thinking would have us be. Perhaps this is what many of us still believe, deep down?

- **Viewing Point 2:** Sex is driven by a relentless desire for pleasure and satisfaction, the pursuit of fun and enjoyment. Well, it is certainly wonderfully delicious and delightful. But the fact that it brings pleasure does not mean that its primary purpose is pleasure.

Excessive obsession with the drive for mere pleasure can easily become a kind of drug, and "the addiction to it is no less profane than actual drug addiction".[95]

Of course the art of love should be pleasurable. This has been part of the ancient lore of the East for centuries, and the accoutrements of high romance in our culture. But there is a vast difference in attitude between the fine art of sensory pleasure and the manic pursuit thereof for various kinds of ego satisfaction.

(Does the desire for pleasure disappear with menopause?)

- **Viewing Point 3:** Sex is a commodity! In this more modern variation, sex is something to have, to get, to do and be done with, like a fast-food product, feeding the ego, not the soul. "Modern lovers

---

"Modern lovers leap into bed and grab ... with gusto as if their bedroom was a fast sex restaurant and their lover an instant orgasm burger in a plain white sack."

leap into bed and grab ... with gusto as if their bedroom was a fast sex restaurant and their lover an instant orgasm burger in a plain white sack."[96]

Have you heard the injunction to "make love as if you are being watched"? What exactly does that mean – sex as performance art? See how sexy I can be! Big ego trip!

(Do you still want to "have" sex?)

- **Viewing Point 4:** Sex is a sin (except in marriage, of course, and then only according to what is "permitted" – all hail the missionary position!)

Why in heaven's name would he, she, they who reside in the higher realms declare this essential, powerful energy a sin? But they do. At least the custodians of the fundamental Judeo-Christian-Islamic religious structures do, where toxic ideas of the essential impurity of sex easily follow notions of the innate sinfulness of women.

In an old Hebrew prayer, a married man prays for forgiveness "for my excesses in the realm of the permitted and my transgressions in the realm of the forbidden. Cleanse me of all impurity."[97] What exactly is unholy and impure here?

An 18th century Christian nun had other ideas; she was a scandalously sensual abbess involved in secret "mystical sensualism"

At least the custodians of the fundamental Judeo-Christian-Islamic religious structures do, where toxic ideas of the essential impurity of sex easily follow notions of the innate sinfulness of women.

practices.⁹⁸ "As our spirit is free, it is only the intention that can make an action wicked. It is enough, therefore, to lift ourselves in our minds up to God, and then nothing is sinful."

The "enjoyment of God" was reached by the act that united one with God, and this was effected "by the cooperation of man and woman, of the man in whom I recognise God". She concluded: "To practice that which we mistakenly call impurity is true purity, which God wishes and bids us to practice and without which we have no way of finding God, who is truth." Basically, through sex we can get to God!

Great nun, this! But clearly the church would have none of her theory.

- **Viewing Point 5:** Sex is an unrelenting need, an incurable everlasting want, compelled by the force of carnal lust, the sins of the brute, un-spiritual, physical flesh, the insistent, urgent, unsatisfied bodily appetite, the longing of (evil) flesh to discharge the tension of "that venereal fury".⁹⁹

As Shakespeare, who had much to say about love and sex, said:

> *The expense of spirit in a waste of shame*
> *Is lust in action; and till action, lust*
> *Is perjur'd, murderous, bloody, full of blame ...*¹⁰⁰

By this definition, maybe, sex is primitive, animalistic – although these words insult the clear purpose of the primitive and the right

---

The "enjoyment of God" was reached by the act that united one with God, and this was effected "by the cooperation of man and woman, of the man in whom I recognise God".

action of the animals. In modern human form it is merely degraded; sex as stress relief of the basest order.

Appetite for coitus is not appetite for love. Are we simply vessels for mutual masturbation, or indeed solo masturbation, on another?

Maybe a good loud scream or punching a pillow would do the same trick, or some hard exercise, a good run, a sweaty workout, or a good body shake all over. How narrow-minded we are in avenues for energy discharge. How we misuse the greatest avenue for big-time energy release – by using it for mere stress release.

Viewing Point 6: Sex is a matter of conjugal duty, a legal and social obligation, because we owe it to our husbands (lords and masters). It is something we have to do, a task on our domestic check list, a job, to get over with, for king and country because of the trouble that happens if we don't, because our mothers said we must, because it's our duty to satisfy his "needs".

Oh boy! Is it any wonder, then, that many married women are actually relieved at the thought that menopause gives them a culturally endorsed reason to forget about IT. They now have a more comprehensive excuse, much better than the periodic headache, to avoid matrimonial duty. Asexual old age, here I come!

Is it any wonder that sex becomes profaned and boring?

Appetite for coitus is not appetite for love. Are we simply vessels for mutual masturbation, or indeed solo masturbation, on another?

- **Viewing Point 7:** "Sex is the greatest magical force in nature," says Evola.[101] It is metaphysical in nature.

All of us will remember some early passionate encounter when the promise of love evoked such a deep yearning for sublime union that it felt like a merging with the very "mystery of the One".

Evola suggests that something of this yearning persists "even when almost everything in the relationship between man and woman deteriorates into animal embraces and is exhausted and dispersed in a faded idealizing sentimentality or in the habitual routine of socially acceptable conjugal relations":

"... if any reflection of a transcendence actually experienced unintentionally takes form in ordinary existence, it does so through sex, and, in the case of the common man, through sex alone."[102]

What, then, is our viewing point on sex – this inherent energy we take so much for granted? To choose a viewing point is to choose our symbolic framework. Our lens of perception determines our experience; we choose our metaphor, and it lives us as the subtle bridge between spirit and matter.

The way we choose to see sex, our metaphoric vehicle, will influence the ride we have.

If sex for us means only the primitive, physical, or profane, we are

---

All of us will remember some early passionate encounter when the promise of love evoked such a deep yearning for sublime union that it felt like a merging with the very "mystery of the One".

carnally afflicted. The affliction lies in our self-chosen viewing point – our metaphor. I will understand when we are glad that it's over; when our decaying bodies give us the ultimate excuse. We will have chosen to give up on the real magic.

The affliction lies in our self-chosen viewing point – our metaphor.

4.3 SACRED CEREMONY & RITUAL UNION

The profound metaphysical aspect of sex was manifest historically in ancient, pagan, and foreign civilisations where sexuality was understood in radically different ways to our limited individualistic and private experience.

Sexual energy was a sacred force that influenced the cosmos, the community, and the earth. The physical union was the symbolic mechanism for elevated processes and purposes: for public religious purposes, for fertility and harvest, for invocation, for initiation, for magic, for blessing the community and protecting the social order through many secret erotic forms and strange rituals that arouse and titillate the profane imagination.

This tantalising world of holy, sacred sexual rites is widely unknown in our popular modern culture, and where known, is often kept secret or dismissed as pagan or evil. Visions of un-holy Dionysian orgies we cannot understand. Horror at the alleged sexual rites of the poor witches of medieval Europe probably had the most to do with their cruel demise.

It is safe to say this kind of stuff freaks out conventional minds. But please stay with me here. Why am I telling you all this? Why should you know this stuff?

Because appreciating the symbolic "magic" of sexual energy as expressed in sexual practices of the past expands our perspective, as

---

Sexual energy was a sacred force that influenced the cosmos, the community, and the earth.

well as our appreciation of this most "basic" energy that we think we know – and all have access to. It can inspire us to re-imagine and respect our sexuality in a different way.

I am not proposing that we copy rites and rituals that applied to different cultures and social milieus. I am suggesting that we review the meaning of our sexuality, its tremendous potential, its profound nature – and the constraints of our profaned perspective.

As Westerners, we emphasize the pure and private experience, rather than symbolic purposes or public display. But unless our imaginations can encompass the astounding nature of sexual energy, we risk trivialising its place and potency within our private lives – and trivialising our lives.

Ritual sexual union was a sacrament to evoke the divine union of the male and female principle outside of time and space, whether as Holy Marriage of King and Queen, God and Goddess, or everlasting Cosmic or Absolute Man and Cosmic or Absolute Woman.

Variations of these holy unions are found in all cultures. Before the Christian era there were mystery rites in Egyptian, Indian, and Greek mythology, including the strange stories of the Eleusinian mysteries. During the Common Era there were sexual rituals for initiation into special societies, or to higher levels of consciousness, as in Hermetic and Western practices of sexual magic.

I am suggesting that we review the meaning of our sexuality, its tremendous potential, its profound nature – and the constraints of our profaned perspective.

"For the Kabbala, every true wedding was in fact a symbolic recreation of the union of God with the Shekhinah."[103]

Wherever family was deemed a holy institution, sexuality was consecrated within that framework. Marriage was about families, clans, dynasties – the social order – rather than individual experience! Arranged marriages make sense in this context – not much room for personal love there. This applied most especially to the women's mothering role as bearer of the lineage, the holy blood line of each family. (This overtly separates the erotic from the child-bearing role, opening up concubinage and multiple wives, but that's another story.)

Control of the sexual energy in our world is now vested in our religions and our governments, who have officially sanctioned the procreative act within marriage – and reproduction is legalized there. Although modern marriage may still aspire to be holy, its mystery is somewhat desecrated.

Another sacrament, that of sacred prostitution, goes way back to the goddess days of the ancient Mediterranean and Far East. It was as different to profane prostitution as the holy Catholic Eucharist wine is to cheap plonk on a drunken Saturday night, and similar in function and intent – a holy, ceremonial, symbolic evocation or worship of the divine presences, however defined.

The sacred prostitute was the priestess of the goddess, whom she

---

Although modern marriage may still aspire to be holy, its mystery is somewhat desecrated.

embodied, and in whose honour she was worshipped, and in whose temples she presided. "These young women, called virgins, pure ones, or blessed ones, were deemed to embody the goddess and to be bearers of the goddess, in their specifically erotic duty." [104]

The patriarchy obviously killed this off long ago, calling her carnal and profane. But ceremonial copulation with the goddess was, for the men involved, a virtue, a prayer, a sacrament. Ritual sex was the very channel for his participation in goddess worship.

It might even be that the ritual postures of the ancient arts of love are the diluted legacy of the priestesses' ancient sacred sexual wisdom of the highest, most subtle resonance, long-lost practices that transformed sensual sex into the super-sensual, psychic, and holy. So much is lost in time and legend!

Basically, men would go to the temple to worship naked women as the living goddess with ancient rites that culminated in sex. Furthermore, young women would have to go to the temple for formal initiation into sex, before they could go home and marry normally. Our limited imagination finds this hard to hold, applying a pornographic interpretation to something that was profound respect of the highest order.

Personally, I am perfectly happy these days with sex as a private experience, rather than communal display. But the idea of ritualized initiation might have a place in the modern world, where teenagers

---

Our limited imagination finds this hard to hold, applying a pornographic interpretation to something that was profound respect of the highest order.

who know nothing rut around mindlessly. Clearly our methods are not working. Even those virginal couples who come together for the first time in marriage fumble around for too long. Sexual education is one thing; proper initiation another, whatever that might mean today.

Sexual education is one thing; proper initiation another, whatever that might mean today.

4.4 VITALITY, HEALTH & LONGEVITY

The general consensus today tells us that sex is good for our health, like fresh fruit and vegetables and a good night's sleep.

But sex is actually exceedingly good for our health; the ancient Chinese Taoist adepts knew that a long time ago, and developed a whole science for achieving vitality, longevity, and health using sexual energy. Sex was overtly part of medicinal healing; the conserving and transforming of sexual energy was a tonic for one's general health.

Their secret of circulating sexual energy along certain pathways inside the body has been passed down for thousands of years in China (and in the Yoga and Tantra traditions of India), where it brought extraordinary improvements in health.

The Taoists worked with breath and with energy channels in the body – conceptually analogous to the wiring of a house, but without real wires. Like an imaginary magnetic circuit, mental not metal. If it sounds psychosomatic, well, it is. We use our imagination, attention, and inner sensation. If it sounds like meditation, well, it is that also. Sex as meditation – another new idea for the West!

South American shamans teach similar concepts – about a fire breath which circulates sexual energy through the body – for health and vitality. The currents of energy are activated in the pelvic area and then mentally directed to successively higher energy centres of the body.

But sex is actually exceedingly good for our health; the ancient Chinese Taoist adepts knew that a long time ago, and developed a whole science for achieving vitality, longevity, and health using sexual energy.

The point to remember here is simply this – they are talking about motions of energy, internal winds, and fires; they are not discussing genital hots and ejaculation!

A less attractive, misogynist part of this tradition involved men stealing sexual energy from women, and, in a parallel practice, Chinese female initiates leeched from the men. Such unfortunate ideas also appear in aspects of what was called Western sexual magic. I mention them only for the sake of thoroughness; they are patriarchal maladaptations of powerful secrets.

The Taoist and Tantric techniques have become available in the West and adapted in a less misogynist manner, with men and women sharing energy, exchanging energy, rather than stealing from each other. There are books that describe very specific ways to direct energy to heal organs, bones, blood, and glands for general vitality,[105] as well as exercises to increase one's sexual health and strength - with a partner or alone.

Such are the health benefits of the very same sexual energy that is used for bad, sad, and dutiful sex, mundane and profane, love and lust – the sublime and the sacred! And this is that same sexual energy that some simply shut down because there is no one to "have" sex with - the confusion of "sexually active" and an active sexuality.

The point to remember here is simply this – they are talking about motions of energy, internal winds, and fires; they are not discussing genital hots and ejaculation!

4.5 EROS & ECSTACY: GETTING HIGH ON SEX

Sex can be transcendent – a bridge to super-consciousness, ecstatic trance, and higher realms – a non-drug-induced, altered state of consciousness. In modern language, we can get high on sex!

What is this "higher intoxication" — this non-physical, metaphysical intoxication, that doesn't loose its quality in the "spasm"?[106]

When we get high on sex, what are we getting high on? When we feel deep sexual attraction, erotic longing, and passionate desire, for what are we yearning? When we merge with our beloved, into what energy do we desire so deeply to melt?

Eros, from whom derives the word erotic, is the love god in Greek mythology, whose arrow pierces our hearts and compels us to fall in love despite ourselves. The desire is overwhelming, having the character of a divine force, a power from beyond rational or ego control.

The symbolism of the Eros story in Western culture points to the higher nature of the sexual energy; Eros as a god-force, a force of nature, like gravity, like light, like the electromagnetic field between positive and negative poles – an irresistible force of attraction. Sexual intercourse is the mechanism of Eros – a resonant electromagnetic coupling.

Eros is now defined as "the sum total of the life preserving and self

---

Eros as a god-force, a force of nature, like gravity, like light, like the electromagnetic field between positive and negative poles – an irresistible force of attraction.

preserving instincts, the libido – and opposed to the death instinct".[107] By general definition, then, Eros is the primary psychic driving power, the life force itself. And it is erotic; it is sexual.

"Sexual love is the most universal form of man's obscure search to eliminate duality for a short while, to existentially overcome the boundary between ego and non-ego, between self and not-self," says Evola.[108] Do you really think he is talking about the genital jiggles here, or the release or relief of tension?

If your concept of a human being is simply "biological and naturalistic", then have a beer, have a fuck, have some fun, do your duty, get release. In this way we buy into the "the illusory and uncertain nature of immediate sexual satisfaction" which substitutes for "the realisation of absolute being".[109]

To explore and experience the "liberating ecstasy", we have to fundamentally change our attitudes, beliefs – and our lifestyle. We have to conceive of ourselves and our bodies themselves as being part of spirit and soul: sexuality as an integral part of spiritual life and practices. Flesh and sex become the very tools by which we can ecstatically approximate the experience of unity; unity with our dearly beloved, unity with spirit, soul, the other. Holy bliss! This is big stuff here. This is the God-stuff here. In my flesh I see God, said Job.[110] Now sex becomes an act of devotion and exultation, and a vehicle of prayer; a technique to attain ecstasy. "With my body, I thee worship," once an essential element in Christian mar-

---

This is big stuff here. This is the God-stuff here. In my flesh I see God, said Job.

riage vows, was banned by the Puritans and remains controversial. "When we embrace God with the love of our bodies, the contact is sexual as well as spiritual." [111]

Sexual love can generate physical life – the human child : and sexual love can generate a spiritual life - "the realisation of our absolute being". The language of human love and the language of mystical love, even ascetic mysticism, are profoundly similar, expressing the same exalted erotic yearning – oscillations of the same desire, longing to cohere with the object of love.

In Western philosophic tradition, love was held to be the dominating and motivating force within the universe. The union of lover and beloved was compared to the ultimate goal of all creation: "a union with the sublime goodness and intellect that are contained within God. A 'circle of love' is thus formed between the universe and its creator in which all things find sustenance and fulfilment." [112]

So many loves to intoxicate us, some of them ambivalent. There is romantic love, love of soul, cosmic love, and universal love, love of God, love of friends, of spouse, of parents, of children. Love of humankind, love of nature, love of body, love of life, of your country, your sports team, books and art and chess. There is love of self and of "Self", love of ego, of control, of cruelty, of power. Which love do we serve? Which love does our relationship serve? Which love does our sexuality serve? What takes us up can also take us down. Which High do we get high on? Which Eros do we serve?

The language of human love and the language of mystical love, even ascetic mysticism, are profoundly similar, expressing the same exalted erotic yearning ...

4.6 COSMIC ENERGY & QUANTUM SEX

We have come a long way from the purely physical and the purely genital. Although, let me be clear, I definitely include the physical (somatic) and the genital – but a physical that is deeply felt as body temple imbued with soul, not as evil Eve, messy material; and genitals which are deeply respected, honoured, and activated – divine Yonis, no longer the sewer with passive plumbing!

In the Western world, the transcendent aspect of sex is reflected in the divine force of erotic energy expressed as Eros, the god of love.

Perhaps the mythological images of Eros and Aphrodite, the goddess of love, are insufficient for imaginations unschooled in classical Greek or Jungian psychology. But there are other metaphors for erotic energy – from the Eastern esoteric traditions and, surprisingly, from the cutting edge of modern science, that can help us transmute our sexuality.

In Yoga/Tantra tradition, one universal truth binds all; the macrocosmic body of the universe is reflected in the microcosmic body of the individual through complex energy systems.

Rooted in the subtle (invisible energy) body within and around each of us lies the dazzling life force of a coiled serpent slumbering at the base of the spine – the kundalini.

When this latent power is awakened, it uncoils itself in waves of

---

But there are other metaphors for erotic energy – from the Eastern esoteric traditions and, surprisingly, from the cutting edge of modern science, that can help us transmute our sexuality.

ecstasy and vital currents that ascend through the central channel of the subtle body, and up and down two side channels on either side of the spine, creating a transcendent experience of energies moving in wave frequencies within the physical structure – up to the brain and beyond, to the universal oneness.

"Expansion and contraction are the two main factors that bring one to the high experience of sexual climax, and are at the beginning and end of all creation,"[113] says Yoga and Tantra.

The purpose of Taoist life is to be one with the Tao, the absolute source, "the indescribable sum and absolute source of these energies, which manifest in ever changing form".[114]

The Taoist universe is filled with different kinds of dynamic energy, and the purpose of a conscious human life is to develop the subtle (spiritual) body and balance harmoniously the male/female polarity – yin and yang. It is only by transforming sex energy into spirit – with or without a partner – that one is able to increase one's available energy (for health) and experience pure consciousness (for spirit).

This is achieved by various techniques of cultivating and circulating sexual energy along (psychosomatic) circuits in the body – not unlike the Tantra route.

Yoga, Tantra and Taoism are physical-metaphysical practices – psychosomatic techniques – for the individual to approach the ex-

---

It is only by transforming sex energy into spirit – with or without a partner – that one is able to increase one's available energy (for health) and experience pure consciousness (for spirit).

perience of the essential oneness of the universe. Sexuality is inherent to these practices, although there are ascetic versions as well.

Now, in the wake of these ancient wisdoms, comes modern quantum physics, presenting the same basic universal oneness. Matter, it tells us, is subtly interconnected with other matter in the universe; the spherical wave structure of matter interacts with all the other matter in the universe.

"We cannot decompose the world into independently existing smallest units. As we penetrate into matter, nature does not show us any isolated 'basic building blocks', but rather appears as a complicated web of relations between the various parts of the whole," says master physicist Fritjof Capra.[115]

Infinite and eternal space exists as a wave-medium and contains wave-motions, they say. Matter exists as the spherical wave motion of space, with in-and-out waves. Space is a wave-medium – we are a wave medium – that propagates wave motions. It is all energy; it is all waves! The universe is a pattern of vibration – like the waves of an uncoiled serpent, I say.

"Sex is the life wave, the power of achievement, the force of evolution and transcendence," says Tantra.[116]

"Sexual union itself is a microcosm of the larger subtle energy fields of the universe, and the body itself, is the vessel of transformation," says Taoism.

"Sexual union itself is a microcosm of the larger subtle energy fields of the universe, and the body itself, is the vessel of transformation," says Taoism.

Quantum physics does not propose a sexual practice, but it discusses "resonant coupling" as a cause of light. What does that sound like?

"We are, in our essential makeup, composed of the same stuff and held together by the same dynamics as those which account for everything else in the universe."[117] We are waves of energy and the whole universe is a vibrating dance of quantum waves and energy exchange. Matter is energy; energy is spirit; spirit is the universe. Energy is matter; consciousness and energy are one.

This then is the nature of our quantum wave world. This is the language of science today. Is it science? Is it metaphysics? Is it sex?

In this way individual consciousness is linked with infinite consciousness, and sexual energy becomes metaphysical, psychic, cosmic. How can we any longer cling to the view of body as simply physical, rather than part of the body/mind/spirit/soul/cosmic/ continuum?

The world IS erotic because the life force itself is erotic, because everything that is sensual and physical also has a spiritual resonance. The life force spiritualizes matter. Matter contains the cosmos; psyche and soma are linked.

The edge of science today offers us this mind-altering metaphor, and image of life and truth, that we can apply to our sexuality – as well as our psychology.

The wave images of quantum physics can be used as the transform-

---

The edge of science today offers us this mind-altering metaphor, and image of life and truth, that we can apply to our sexuality – as well as our psychology.

ing image of quantum sex. We said earlier that when sexuality and spirituality were split in our culture "we lost contact with what unites them". Here, in the language of science, is the missing link that unifies it all – the universal in-and-out waves. It is all one.

With this metaphor, what becomes the nature of the sexual union – of our sexuality? And what have we been doing our whole life? What will we do for the rest of it?

In sex, we activate the standing waves of the universe inside of us, carried on the winds and fluids within our bodies.

In sex, the waves of the universe vibrate in us. The streaming sensations we feel in our physical form are also the wave energies of the universe. This may sound like an unattainable, perhaps fictional, ideal. But I believe it is so, and that we – and that means you – can become conscious of it, to our incalculable benefit.

When we surrender to orgasm, we allow ourselves to vibrate in the universe. Every sensation, thought, and emotion becomes saturated with holy bliss. "Inside of you is what is outside of you,"[118] says the old oracle.

The psychosomatic energy that circulates is universal energy. At the root of sex we discover the cosmos; the mysterious centre of spirituality hides an erotic heart. Our physical matter is holy. Holy bliss indeed!

In sex, we activate the standing waves of the universe inside of us, carried on the winds and fluids within our bodies.

This is quantum sex – the new/old sacred sex for the post-menopausal years.

It can work alone – or with a beloved partner. It can work with much physical effort or with little. No more mutual masturbation; now it's mutual divine meditation – experiencing the divinity of the partner!

Quantum sex! And we want to be finished with the whole messy business?

Like waves from water, flames from fire and rays from the sun, the waves of the universe differentiate out from what? Are we talking God; or the Tao, Shiva/Shakti, Great Spirit – or quantum physics?

Matter and energy in science parallel Shakti and Shiva in Tantra, Ida and Pingala in Yoga, yin and yang in Taoism. All of these are metaphors for body and spirit, carrying positive and negative force. They need to be in delicate balance – not hierarchical. No superior / inferior here. No sinful flesh. No matter mattering less than spirit.

Sexual union becomes a symbolic act of "imitatio dei", imitation of God – experiencing the divinity of the partner. But there has been a problem here for too long; the divine in man requires an equivalent divine woman – not one debased, demeaned, or devalued.

The god needs his goddess – and the goddess needs to be just that. But in our world they killed the Great Goddess, and blamed Eve

---

Sexual union becomes a symbolic act of "imitatio dei", imitation of God – experiencing the divinity of the partner.

for everything "wrong" with woman. Patriarchy and its accompanying misogyny hurt men and women alike – most especially in our sexuality.

We need to redeem the goddess within. Ironically, we cannot do that without also redeeming post-menopausal women. Because the Goddess has three parts, as we will see in the next section – and, of the three, the old Crone had the worst time of all. Although she embodied the archetype of wisewoman, she was repressed and reviled, crippling all women together with the Crone.

Quantum sex requires empowered women who have redeemed the goddess within, which means, among other self-loving things, liberating the mythological Crone – and her wisdom – and her sexuality.

Whither the old woman then, whither the witch? A quantum challenge indeed.

Patriarchy and its accompanying misogyny hurt men and women alike – most especially in our sexuality.

CHAPTER 5
TOWARDS A NEW "OLD" AGE

The bleak stereotypes we examined earlier simply don't serve us any more. They are caricatures, reflecting the historically inferior status of women and the suppression of the Goddess. Dare we re-imagine, indeed invent, admirable new prototypes of being – new myths to live by?

5.1 GODDESS METAPHORS & THE HEKATE PROBLEM

By definition, a stereotype is an unjustifiably fixed and standardized mental image – often unkind and untrue as well.[119] Archetypes are alive, fluid, primordial mental images that are ever present in the collective unconscious. They pump vitality into life. Stereotypes are rigid and dead, and they parody archetypes.

Archetypes are the "magnetic energy field" at the core of personal psychological issues; the grand archetype of "mother", for instance, as distinct from our personal mother and mothering. But mother is only one aspect of our being – overwhelming though she is.

Where are inspirational mythological images of being older and female? There is no authoritative manual of new myths to live by. Our very lives today are the testing ground for new prototypes of being post-menopausal.

The closest we come is Jean Shinoda Bolen's Goddesses in Older Women: archetypes in women over fifty. (This and her previous book, Goddesses in Everywoman, are without a doubt required reading for conscious women living today, as is Marion Woodman's Dancing in the Flames.)

Each of the Greek goddesses she describes represents a different archetype operating in our psyche. Where we are most identified with the traditional roles of wife, mother, or daughter, we are metaphori-

---

Where are inspirational mythological images of being older and female? There is no authoritative manual of new myths to live by.

cally living out Hera, the goddess of marriage and archetypical wife; Demeter, archetypical mother or Persephone, the maiden goddess and queen of the underworld (the eternal girl and inner guide), respectively.

Our autonomous qualities are aspects of the virginal Artemis, goddess of the hunt and moon (sister, feminist, goal achiever); Athena, goddess of wisdom and crafts (strategist, warrior, craftswoman); and Hestia of the hearth and temple (anonymous woman, hearth keeper).

Love, sexuality, and beauty are the domain of sensuous Aphrodite (lover, creative woman). She is the goddess mother of Eros, and like his, her force is magnetic and compulsive.

But where are the post-menopausal goddesses?

In Goddesses in Older Women, Bolen has to scratch around to find venerable older goddesses. The only "older" woman in the Greek stories is the "dimly seen" Hekate, goddess of the crossroads who could see three ways at once.[120] She is the "goddess at the threshold of major transitions", the midwife at birth – and at death, representing intuition and psychic wisdom.

None of the other older-goddess archetypes that Bolen presents are intrinsically old. She gathers them across diverse religions and cultures, to mirror real-life issues of contemporary older women who are consciously exploring their post-menopausal years for "wisdom, compassion, active action, and healing humour".

But where are the post-menopausal goddesses?

In order to describe mystical and spiritual wisdom, Bolen uses the hidden Christian Sophia, who, like the exiled Jewish Shekhina, is the feminine face of God. There is the practical and intellectual Metis (the miniaturized Titan goddess swallowed by a fearful Zeus), and the meditative Hestia; the fierce Egyptian Sekhmet and Hindu Kali express wrath and outrage; Greek Baubo and the Japanese Uzume heal with laughter; and the Chinese Kuan Yin, the Virgin Mary, and America's Lady Liberty symbolize kindness and compassion.

Patriarchy diminished or demonized most of these goddess attributes, and the general sense of a sacred, powerful feminine was lost. (The Greek goddesses themselves were merely split remnants of the Great Goddess, long conquered by the patriarchal pantheon. Ancient Greece was good to its men only; women were the property of men, and could own none in their own right.)

Aphrodite was demoted to goddess of harlots; "good" women had a hard time identifying with her without guilt. The Hera wife was typecast as jealous and vengeful, when she really yearned for a sacred marriage, "to be in spiritual, emotional and physical union in which the intimacy ... is experienced by both as sacred".[121]

The wise, psychic, and reclusive Hecate became witch and old hag; like all "the grey-haired high priestesses, once respected tribal matriarchs of pre-Christian Europe", she was transformed into the devil's consort.[122] Like Lilith, she was rejected, feared, and left to wander the wilderness in dark twilight shadows, a spiritual outcast.

Without a sacred feminine, there is no place for a Divine Old Woman – only witches and hags, sweet grannies and menopausal madness. And no place for sacred sex, either!

The archetypes who fared the worst were wife, lover, and old woman – wives were owned, sex was bad with a few exceptions, and female wisdom was reviled or denied. No wonder the lives of real older women were/are so constrained, with the result that there are few admirable role models of older women in past centuries – and in recent times.

Without a sacred feminine, there is no place for a Divine Old Woman – only witches and hags, sweet grannies and menopausal madness. And no place for sacred sex, either!

Long ago, in pre-patriarchal times, older wise women were priestesses, initiators, ceremonial leaders, midwives, healers, teachers, spiritual advisors, prophets, funerary officials. But old women in Europe were stripped of their wise-woman status when the newly established universities of the 11th century officially excluded women, and public service required proper credentials.

What female healers remained by the 14th century were targeted by the church. "If any women cured sickness without having studied medicine at a university, she was a witch and must die."[123] The "old" medicine wisdom of women healers and midwives was reduced to "old wives' tales". Every 'witch' way, older women were marginalized.

The mysterious Hekate was wise like Sophia; it is hidden in the name itself. (Wisdom in Hebrew is Hok-mah.) But the patriarchy feared this wisdom – calling it witchcraft. What was this mysterious witchcraft they feared so much? The healing skills of a doctor,

---

But old women in Europe were stripped of their wise-woman status when the newly established universities of the 11th century officially excluded women, and public service required proper credentials.

intuitive knowledge of a sage, dream expertise of a Jungian therapist, prophesy of a seer, herbal knowledge of an alchemist, manifestation techniques of a shaman, conjuring skills of a magician?

Hekate was there at the crossroads of death and birth – in some ways a feminine version of the bearded wise old man who lived in the sky. Except that in the patriarchal universe there was no place for a divinely wise old woman in the sky – or on earth. She had to be rejected – and with her, old women generally.

Hekate was barely seen; she had only brief cameo roles in the Greek dramas. For the rest she was invisible – as old women in our society have become. In popular imagination she was witch and the wicked stepmother of fairy tales; clever but terrible.

Nancy Friday writes that "older women were once seen as witches because of their power; it was the older woman's embodiment of sexual energy, not her dried-up old sex that frightened men and other women too, who were not so emboldened."[124] Riding on a broomstick, indeed! The broom handle is the phallus?

But there was no social container in a patriarchal world to live such a reality, since she was no longer wife nor mother nor maiden. Was Hekate asexual or "dangerously" sexual? What does "dangerously

---

> "...older women were once seen as witches because of their power; it was the older woman's embodiment of sexual energy, not her dried-up old sex that frightened men and other women too, who were not so emboldened. Riding on a broomstick, indeed! The broom handle is the phallus?"

sexual" mean, anyway? Covert knowledge of ancient secrets, maybe.

I like to imagine that Hekate was a beautiful wise old woman with long silver hair and piercing grey eyes who had a secret sexual life when she wasn't combing the crossroads or attending to births and deaths. She had a consort at home, a beloved wise man named Hektor. Perhaps he cooked while she was doing her duties. At home, late at night she would change her black cape for a colourful caftan and exotic makeup. They would light candles and love and laugh at the splendour and fun of their secret (and sexual) lives while everyone else was terrified. We just don't know.

I like to think that Hekate was too wise to be miserable and alone while she waited out the darkness of the patriarchy. "What the heck," she thought – and made the best of it, hiding her brilliance. Well, Hekate, your time has come – the patriarchy is over. What are your secrets?

Well, Hekate, your time has come – the patriarchy is over. What are your secrets?

5.2 RECLAIMING THE CRONE

In legend, the Great Goddess has three aspects – all parts divine; like the moon in her phases, like life itself – past/present/future, birth/life/death. She is Virgin / Mother / Crone; Creatrix / Preserver / Destroyer; Maiden / Wife /Witch.

Other versions describe four aspects; chaste, promiscuous, motherly and bloodthirsty; modest, sensual, nurturing and ruthless; virginal, harlot, fertile and warlike; immaculate, wanton, motherly and warrior.[125]

All renditions have the fierce component and the nurturing/fertile aspect. But sexuality is befuddled and divided; what does it mean to be chaste and promiscuous? We do not have an image for it because our worldview denies a sacred sexuality, sex is either good or bad. So chaste is split from promiscuous, modest from sensual, virgin from harlot, immaculate from wanton.

Essentially the lover aspect is separated from both mother and maiden – and severely condemned. In truth the lover aspect is the priestess of love – serving Eros. She is ecstatic and transcendent in nature. The lover archetype was and should be part of our virgin life, our mother/wife life, and our crone life. (Sacred) sexuality imbues all aspects of the life cycle.

Defining the Virgin by her unbroken hymen is a patriarchal concept, a limited and literal understanding of virginity. Metaphorically and

---

The lover archetype was and should be part of our virgin life, our mother/wife life, and our crone life. (Sacred) sexuality imbues all aspects of the life cycle.

psychologically, the Virgin is the autonomous part of a woman's psyche; the intrinsic self not owned by, needing, or requiring a man's validation. She could be sexual - or not.

(On the matter of "losing your virginity", there is the wonderful story in the novel Red Tent,[126] where the older women gently pierce the hymen at first menstruation with one of those little goddess figurines. Essentially, the menstruating girl's initial physical penetration is an initiation by the goddess – not a male violation with blood on the sheet in barbaric proof of possession.)

The patriarchy had to wrest control of the life cycle from the Goddess. Life and death were fairly straightforward; but to command procreation, the mother/wife had to be owned in marriage, and sexuality had to be strictly confined there. The mother image was even reconfigured to being ever caring and self-effacing – denying her sexual and destructive sides.

By severe distortion, then, the Virgin and Mother phases of the ancient goddess could be assimilated into Christianity. But the Crone absolutely could not; the word itself derives from the word crown, and indicates the lost power of ancient queens. The Crone was wise, mysterious, independent – and awesome. Too much like the male god aspect! According to Barbara Walker,[127] patriarchal religions could not achieve full control of men's minds until the crone figure was suppressed.

By severe distortion, then, the Virgin and Mother phases of the ancient goddess could be assimilated into Christianity. But the Crone absolutely could not ...

Compare the wisdom figure of India, where the divine Shakti is "an almost untranslatable amalgam of wife, mistress, queen, power, genius, strength, authority, mind, vulva, woman and cosmic energy",[128] and every god needed his Shakti in order to act. Here are multifaceted options for real women!

But in the West they crippled our Crone, leaving only images of ugly witches, evil stepmothers, and harmless little old ladies. A wise and wonderful (and sexual) Crone has been absent from our culture and our conscious awareness for too long. Without her, our life options are distorted – and old age bleak indeed.

How do we live as wise (and sexual) crones today, standing in our own experiences? How do we rehabilitate the archetype of the wisewoman? How do we live real lives as contemporary Hekates?

The answer lies in our psychological and spiritual life – first and foremost; the work of soul.

It is only in the work of consciousness that we can free ourselves and our inner Crone. It is our life task to find our relationship to the goddess in all her spheres, as a conscious virgin, mother, and crone.

The crone challenges us to go beyond duality and ego to a both/and world, of psyche and soma – a more conscious world that contains opposites. She calls us to consciousness.

The old matriarchy projected everything outside onto Mother Nature:

It is our life task to find our relationship to the goddess in all her spheres, as a conscious virgin, mother, and crone.

and the patriarchy onto a spiritual father sun. Today "we are moving towards the realisation of an interiorised spirituality," says Marion Woodman,[129] that is like the kingdom within according to Christ, like the higher levels of consciousness of the esoteric traditions of the east, and the individuated Self of modern psychological consciousness.

In this new place we can live from an internal centre, where holding the paradox feeds our transformation and is the passage through. In this place we are penetrated with spirit and we are embodied in our flesh. Imagine being able to simultaneously contain body and mind, good and bad, psyche and soma, masculine and feminine, sex and spirit, and being enriched by this...

By remaining present to the paradox and the inner processes it provokes, we can ground the cosmic in the dark matter of our somatic bodies. This is the duality dance; the core of wisdom; the perpetual cycle of regeneration and transformation.

There are fairy tales of the old hag who transforms into a beautiful young maiden at will. "What a woman desires above all else is the power of sovereignty – the right to exercise her own will." When the knight Gawain kissed the ugly old lady who had told him this life-saving secret she became young and beautiful.[130] The terrifying Kali would sometimes appear as a young maiden; she destroys and redeems the universe as divine mother – and sexual consort.

The Crone's liberation is to "exercise her own will", after centuries, to

---

In this place we are penetrated with spirit and we are embodied in our flesh.

incorporate all aspects, virgin, mother, crone – and lover. In our maturing, our Virgin soul (our princess in the tower) moves to the Crone's wholeness. The Virgin in the hag; the Virgin IS the hag.

Reclaiming the Crone means the spiritual and psychological deepening of soul that maturity can bring, if one does one's personal psychological and spiritual work. It is also the only proper platform for the redefinition of sexuality required at menopause.

Post-menopausal time is the time to live the more transcendental aspects of sex. Having "done" the sexual revolution of the 1960s is not enough. The real and genuine sexual revolution – the endgame of the liberation, is sacred sexuality with a genuine feminine consciousness.

Let menopause be the death of the bad, sad, and dutiful sex – but not the death of sex. In old age, being our authentic selves (in or out of relationship), our sexuality, and our spirituality is the path itself. The reawakening of spirituality and a renewed sexuality are mutually inclusive. It is Crone's work and part of our conscious evolution.

The reawakening of spirituality and a renewed sexuality are mutually inclusive. It is Crone's work and part of our conscious evolution.

5.3 LIVING IN A QUANTUM WORLD

Modern physics once again provides the illuminating metaphor we need to live consciously, spiritually, sexually – even into old age. The feminine, immanent aspect of god/spirit/life – what we call the Goddess – is quantum in nature, and the calling of our time is to bridge the metaphorical gap between psyche and soma.

Our universe is uncertain and full of paradox; the absolutes of good and evil no longer hold. Quantum science describes phenomena as acausal, nonrational, related, non-local, chaotic, complementary, indeterminate. All these are notions associated with femininity in writing and literature. The Goddess IS quantum.

Like the old oracle ... "I am the substance and the one who has no substance".

> *I am the abiding and I am the dissolution*
> *I am the one below*
> *And they come up to me*
> *I am the judgement and the acquittal*
> *I, I am sinless*
> *And the root of sin derives from me.*[131]

The uncertainty inherent in the state of physical matter mirrors our psychic lives, mirrors the universe itself. These things are not mutually exclusive, says quantum physics – indeed they are all absolutely required.

The feminine, immanent aspect of god/spirit/life – what we call the Goddess – is quantum in nature, and the calling of our time is to bridge the metaphorical gap between psyche and soma.

The new physics has a mystical resonance: "The world is a spiritual unity, a dance between soul and spirit – the same dance that scientists find under their microscopes and in their mathematical formulas. Our ancestors were correct in recognising the world as spiritual, but at their stage of development, were able to express this recognition only concretely. Patriarchy, in its turn, has been no more able to go beyond the concrete."[132]

The answer is "neither the undifferentiated world of early matriarchy nor the overly differentiated world of patriarchy."[133] Neither in body, nor in mind, neither in matter, nor in spirit, but in the perpetual dance in-between! The duality dance again.

The connector is soul: the subtle body (otherwise called the light body, the energy body, the metaphorical body); psychologists, poets, and philosophers cannot pin down this thing that scientists cannot measure, but people know to be real. This mid ground between spirit and body is part heaven and part earth.

Here the darkest matter of our body is conscious and sacred, and the divine comes into time and space. This is Woodman's "interiorised spirituality", the arena of psycho-spiritual work today. As "we recognise the non materiality of the body, of nature, the more conscious it becomes. The consciousness is what we call soul, a soul no longer forced into exile."[134]

"Seeing ourselves in this way allows us to act both within ourselves

---

The new physics has a mystical resonance: "The world is a spiritual unity, a dance between soul and spirit – the same dance that scientists find under their microscopes and in their mathematical formulas move.

and within the universe in a manner impossible or inconceivable to earlier generations. A higher level of consciousness is required for such a world view." [135]

Quantum consciousness can bridge the metaphorical gap between psyche and soma. It allows the duality to continue its dance - like the perpetual cycle of regeneration and transformation, like the Crone. Everything seems to come together here. The new understanding of the psychology of the crone, of sexual and cosmic energy, of quantum reality, and of our lives as real people. Between the old matriarchy and the old patriarchy, we wrestle with a new reality and hope that fundamentalism doesn't quash it all.

This then is the challenge of living in our quantum world today. And in this world, how then should we age – and die?

Everything seems to come together here. The new understanding of the psychology of the crone, of sexual and cosmic energy, of quantum reality, and of our lives as real people.

5.4 DEATH, AGEING & SEXUAL BEAUTY

We live in our body but the body will not stay; we are going to die.

Our ego mind might mourn, fear or accept the fact; our soul might know eternity – or not. We 'only don't know' about death, except that dying has its own way. When we die we die.

The only relevant question, then, is how to live while we do this ageing thing that so sabotages our confidence! In a play or drama, the third act culminates and resolves the dramatic theme –it's the point and purpose of the play. Instead of flowering our individuated selves, many sink into frail desolation, glum consensus: or they pretend that nothing has really changed.

Psychologist James Hollis says we develop only a "provisional personality" [136] during the first half of life; whereas the second half is the time for the deepening consciousness of soul to flourish – or not. So many choose to atrophy (spiritually and sexually) from midlife onwards!

What does a glorious old age look like, in our bodies, in our life?

We fear ageing and we fear the ageing body. The truth is we don't know for sure how we are meant to age, men and women alike. Does the body have to decay and crumble and become ill in order to pass over?

Just how much decrepitude, warts, wrinkles, sunspots, waning strength,

---

We fear ageing and we fear the ageing body.

creaking joints, drooping posture, misshapen form, failing mobility, and fading health, with innumerable medical conditions with horrible names – is absolutely inevitable to becoming older?

How much is the self-fulfilling condition of a medical community with an agenda and a culture so deeply brainwashed by the idea that we have to decay enough, or become ill enough, in order to make the final break from this life, and take the grand journey back to the beyond?

We can only be conscious now. We can live healthily and consciously now – and anticipate, intend, and expect vitality. And hope and pray! We just don't know for sure what would manifest if we didn't expect it to be so bleak.

We ourselves will test the new reality in our own bodies, our attitudes, and our life style – a "deliberate and harmonious" old age; being totally open-minded to, and accepting of, what our bodies present us with – even if 'stuff' happens.

If illness or accident comes, taking our new respect for the psychosomatic, it behoves us to treat it as metaphor (even while being treated) by which we can deepen our spiritual process.

The toughest challenge of all, certainly for women baby boomers, is the matter of sexual beauty and to affirm sexual beauty in the crone image staring her in the mirror.

Death, ageing, and even illness is almost easier to accept: it's sexual

---

The toughest challenge of all, certainly for women baby boomers, is the matter of sexual beauty and to affirm sexual beauty in the crone image staring her in the mirror.

ugliness that defeats us. It was hard enough to adjust our bodies to the media prescriptions of our adolescence and adulthood, but for ageing female bodies, the cultural expectation itself is not pretty at all.

"Aging in women is a process of becoming obscene sexually," wrote feminist Susan Sontag in 1972. "One of the attitudes that punish women most severely is the visceral horror felt at aging female flesh."[137] We are revolted by our own image and "turn from sex with self-disgust, seeing in men's eyes our own revulsion". (As if they age that much better physically!)

The sexual revolution is incomplete until it embraces a sacred sexuality; so, too, the whole feminist opus remains only partial until we embody the crone years with genuine wisdom and enthusiasm, and without sexual repulsion.

Nancy Friday challenges again: "Until the reassuring image of a new generation of women has made the journey into a world of sexual beauty, younger women will watch us cautiously, enviously, until the turf is truly won. Then there will be a stampede, not into old age, but into life ongoing. It is modern women's journey and the enemy is within."[138]

What does mature sexual beauty look like in older women with personal power?

Is it possible, and dare we believe to see it in ourselves – and other ageing women? Or will we call other women witches and whores, as our

---

...so, too, the whole feminist opus remains only partial until we embody the crone years with genuine wisdom and enthusiasm, and without sexual repulsion.

medieval sisters did? When we look in the mirror, are we succumbing to fear of ageing? Has it become worse, even though we are living longer and longer?

We have unravelled the psychic shadows, understood the stereotypes, embraced our biology and divine Yoni; we have opened to full body orgasm and ejaculation; we respect the divine power of sexual energy and understand that life and consciousness are quantum, that quantum sex is spiritual, that crone/mother/virgin is an endless dance of transformation – and yet ...

When we look in the mirror, who and what do we see looking back at us?

> *Mirror, mirror on the wall*
> *I didn't look like that before*
> *I am not fairer than the younger she*
> *That flesh that sags – just isn't me*
> *Yet I am she and she was always me*
> *What is real – what imaginary*
> *Help me help me really see*
> *The infinity of beauty ... in me*

A mirror image is a riddle; it is and isn't there.

We see it before us, but we know that our real flesh and bones don't exist in the lead and the glass. The image is a distortion in the quan-

---

When we look in the mirror, who and what do we see looking back at us?

tum field – and our lens of perception. Do you look like your mother; is the witch in you? And the virgin, mother, crone; wise and powerful, wrathful and loving?

Do you hear the sexual condemnation of the "good" mother because you know a few things, sexually speaking, which she did not? Are you still split between good mother and bad mother? Which mother is in the mirror with you? Kind and cruel! Witch and whore! Cursed and honoured?

Can we be all that – and moral and spiritual as well? And sexual – in every way? Can we reconcile and love it all? Can we see it is also as lovely?[139]

Magic mirror on the wall
Lover, harlot, crone – and all
Forgive all mothers – witches and whores
Adjust the lighting, and you will see
The virgin – dying to be reborn
In the physics of spirit
The observer matters
Perceived and perceived is one

Cosmic mirror of the All
Shifting shapes in cosmic waves
Mirror images are there – not there
Holy whore a goddess be
Immanent in the flesh is she – wisdom and sexuality
Every year winter and every year spring
Age and youth inside my matter – until the matter rests
Let the love in my matter make love to you

> For what is inside of you is what is outside of you
> And the one who fashions you on the outside
> Is the one who shaped the inside of you
> And what you see outside of you
> You see inside of you
> It is visible and it is your garment.[140]

What else can I say? It is your challenge and mine to redeem the crone when we redeem the sexual beauty of the older woman in ourselves.

We do that when we can look in the mirror and smile, and sincerely say – In my flesh I see God, Goddess/All that is – In my flesh I see THEE.

5.5 LIFE ONGOING

> *I am wise and a witch.*
> *I am spiritual and material*
> *I am chaste and gloriously sexual*
> *I am useful and I am lovely*
> *I am your friend, mentor, mother and lover*
> *And the only princess I keep locked in towers*
> *is my own unfinished soul.*

There are no answers here about life ongoing, as I myself have just entered this period. What do I know what is achievable – or not?

It is all too early to say. I am "only" 58 and still "looking good". Who is to know what will unfold? Nevertheless I have made the call.

We are our own daily research project on living a quantum life ongoing – until we go. Life ongoing is the spiritual journey before the hereafter – a real-life exploration of the edges of conscious life.

"Age does not protect you from love. But love, to some extent, protects you from age." [141]

Can we complete the sexual revolution by making sex sacred, feminized, and real in our crone years? Quantum sex! How sad it would be if future historians talked about the 1960s as a temporary liberation only – a brief sexual enlightenment.

We are our own daily research project on living a quantum life ongoing – until we go. Life ongoing is the spiritual journey before the hereafter – a real-life exploration of the edges of conscious life.

Can we dare to imagine and live a sacred marriage with a beautiful wise old man – Hekate and Hektor?

Can we round off the great feminist achievements by living a conscious cronehood that can inspire younger women, rather than terrify?

A manifesto is a public declaration of intentions, motives, or principles of actions. I hope I have done that. I have had to go down various avenues, to support my view that there is a different way. We must be able to separate out the old history, the wrong psychology, the warped anatomy, and the perverted beliefs.

My manifesto is simply this: to live sexually, spiritually, soulfully, and "quantumly" in this wonderful world. To commit to the quantum sex that is intimacy and love of the other, and love of the Self, and Love of the OTHER – call it God, Great Spirit, All that Is ... Our sense of it is overwhelming, our rational understanding of it limited. So what matters what we call it? It is divine and it is sexual and it is forever!

My manifesto is simply this: to live sexually, spiritually, soulfully, and "quantumly" in this wonderful world.

APPENDIX

Relationships

I have specifically excluded any reference to building good relationships, as my focus has been on sexuality. There are certainly enough books and courses out there. However, the subject is implicit, in the sense that I urge psycho-spiritual work to increase consciousness; relationship issues are often addressed in this context. And anyway, the more we become clear on all of our issues, the more we are one with ourselves, the better our relationships become.

Economics of ageing

The large wave of senior citizens from the baby boom generation is considered a looming financial problem for societies that pension people off in their 60s, and where the state is supposed to look after them for ever after. As long as we take the view that old age will inevitably be a time of increasing illness, and as long as the proportion of the relatively young working population is less than the big grey wave, well, yes, huge problems are afoot.

But what if we actually take responsibility for living healthily, looking out for optimum health rather than the least amount of illness and ailments? Would this not be a better world anyway, with a senior community who can still make a difference in our world? Or, at least, be less of a burden.

Healthier old people can also be economically productive, which is an important aspect. We need to re-envision our work life to include work that can be done in later years, as well as the whole concept of finances, pensions, and investments.

Third World women

I am very aware that I have been addressing the older women of the modern Western world. I do, however, want to note and honour the many older women of Africa and other developing economies who are facing a unique and difficult challenge. With a whole generation of young adults decimated by Aids, many older women are bringing up young grandchildren and eking out a living alone and under difficult conditions. I pray for a world where all older women can focus on their spiritual development rather than basic sustenance. I respectfully honour their grit and their courage.

PART TWO
SELF-ASSESSMENT
QUESTIONNAIRE

SELF-ASSESSMENT QUESTIONNAIRE
REVIEW YOUR SEXUAL SELF

1. Are you perfectly comfortable with your genitals? Do you deeply honour and accept your genitalia, without echoes of shame or any embarrassment whatsoever?

    A Only a little
    B No, not at all
    C Yes I am; I deeply honour and accept my most intimate, feminine perfection, especially my genitalia. I can be fully open and surrendered and confident.

2. Do you understand the concept of energy orgasm and energy flows, as distinct from genital focus? Do you understand the concept of being sexually alive, without necessarily having a parner to be "sexually active" with.

    A A little, sort of
    B No I do not
    C I fully understand the metaphysical dimensions of body imbued with soul.

3. Can you imagine that sexuality and spiritually are aspects of the same thing, that the very energy of sex is itself universal energy?

    A No I can't
    B Maybe a little
    C Yes, I can honestly say that I have experienced my sexuality as holy, embodied spirit, inherently divine – and fun.

4 Do you understand the difference between orgasm and ejaculation in women. Have you ever had an ejaculation?

   A Sort of, maybe
   B No I do not; no I have not
   C Yes I do; yes I have and it deepened my experience.

5 Have you in any way within your heart and mind, given up on sex because you have "done" or "are doing" menopause? Do you feel less sexual?? Do you feel less confident about the sexuality that you do feel?

   A Well yes a little
   B Yes a lot
   C Not at all; I feel more sexual in a holistic, mature & ecstatic way. I experience/d menopause as a positive experience of soul, a physical and spiritual gateway to the third phase of my life.

6 Are you afraid of aging? Does the thought of being an older woman arouse vague, uncomfortable ambivalent feelings within you?. Do your mirror reflections tease you with sagging flesh that was once unequivocally firm and ghost images of old women you wish you weren't becoming?

   A Yes a little
   B Yes a lot
   C Not at all; I have a clear vision of aging and I perfectly and joyously accept every facet of my sagging flesh

7   Are you confused about how you should view yourself sexually, now that you are an "older woman"? Do you feel its inappropriate to be sexual now in terms of your previous experience and knowledge?

A   Yes a little
B   Yes a lot
C   Not at all; I have a clear expansive sense of joyous sexual awareness.

RESULTS

Anything less than sincere affirmations of all the number 3 choices, means you still have thoughts, feelings, attitudes and beliefs around the stuff of sexuality to clear; its only a matter of degree.

If most of your answers were no 1, you have a vague idea of a world inside of you that you do not know yet. There are important wisdoms that will only increase your joy in being alive, whether you are in relationship or not.

If most of your answers were no 2, then you really don't know what you don't know. Hurry! There is a fascinating new world awaiting you as you untumble the myths that mess with your joy.

PART THREE
"WORKING WITH MY SEXUALITY"
The Healing Workbook

THE HEALING WORKBOOK

A personal program of reflections, memories, exercises & meditations towards a more soulful sexuality. (These have nothing to do with a partner at this point. Its for everyone.)

This program can be done at your own pace, or you can dedicate a week or a month to each section.

It is best to read Part One of this book before you being the programme, because its information will provide context and help you see beyond the beliefs you have held to be indubitably true - and inspire you to plunge into the truth of your interior beliefs and attitudes.

SECTION 1: UNCOVERING CORE BELIEFS
SECTION 2: RECALLING SEXUAL HISTORY
SECTION 3: MEETING BODY & SOUL
SECTION 4: MAKING NEW CHOICES

1 UNCOVERING MY CORE BELIEF
REFLECT & JOURNAL

Take time to reflect on these questions. Make quiet private time in a good space for yourself. Light a candle if you want, to mark it as sacred self-knowledge time. Dig deep inside your heart, soul and mind. Be honest, no matter how embarrassing the answers. No-one needs see this other than yourself.

YOUR NAME: _____

A   WHAT I REALLY BELIEVE ABOUT SEX

Sex is mainly:

Physical/genital/emotional/mental/spiritual/for procreation/fun/sinful

Circle the ones that resonate with you. Add others.

_____
_____
_____
_____
_____
_____
_____

My best thoughts about sex are:

_____
_____

Write more on a separate sheets if you need to.

My most negative thoughts about sex are :

_____

_____

_____

_____

_____

_____

Reflect on your answers. How do they make you feel?.
Write more on a separate sheets if you need to. You could also draw what you feel – or sing it – or dance it.

B WHAT I REALLY BELIEVE ABOUT MENOPAUSE?

Menopause is mainly:

the end of sex/the end of procreation/an illness/a collection of physical symptoms/psychological depression/mania/a medical experience

Circle the ones that resonate with you. Add others.

My best thoughts about menopause are:

Write more on a separate sheets if you need to.

My most negative thoughts about menopause are:

Reflect on your answers. How do they make you feel?.
Write more on a separate sheets if you need to. You could also draw what you feel – or sing it – or dance it.

B WHAT I REALLY BELIEVE ABOUT AGING WOMEN?

Older women are wise/ worthless/ sweet/ sexual/ asexual/ witches/ ugly /socially useless/powerful/ weak/ oversexed

Circle the ones that resonate with you. Add others.

_____
_____
_____
_____
_____
_____
_____

My best images of older, post menopausal / aging women / are:

_____
_____
_____
_____
_____
_____
_____

Write more on a separate sheets if you need to.

My most negative images of older, post menopausal / aging women are:

_____
_____
_____

_____

_____

_____

_____

Reflect on your answers. How do they make you feel?.
Write more on a separate sheets if you need to. You could also draw what you feel – or sing it – or dance it.

2 RECALLING MY SEXUAL HISTORY

Take the time to go back in time to remember long lost memories and feelings, the good and the bad. Remembering and then releasing is a powerful psycho-spiritual tool of personal growth. Make notes, or journal, or record or simply just contemplate. Take your time – and notice your feelings and thoughts around these memories

MEMORIES

A   REMEMBER THE CHILD

Revisit, in your mind, images of yourself as a child and how and what you were taught about your regarding your sexuality, and mother's, and father's? What you felt, what you feared? What you dared to imagine? Do a bit of stocktaking on the terrible stories you were taught, and imagine their impact on your tender young psyche. Take time to release them.

_____
_____
_____
_____
_____
_____
_____

B   REFLECT THE YOUTH

Reflect on the masturbations of your youth, what you did, how you felt about it. Was it discovered, how did your parents struggle against it or permit it, did you succeed in suppressing it, or rationalising it away? How did these ideas in some way influence your adult sexuality? Acknowledge and grab those thoughts of shame, guilt etc, and re-imagine them in a new light.

C REVIEW THE ADULT

Do a personal recapitulation of your adult sexual experiences: the joys, the highlights and delights, as well as the blind, bland, bumbling, stupid, risqué and ...

Did your sexuality over these years operate from the physical, emotional, mental and spiritual? Which has been the primary aspect? Which the least?

Notice your feelings – all your feelings. Be kind to yourself. Forgive yourself! Release remembered pain and shame. Gently laugh at yourself. Rejoice in the good memories. You can journal if you want, or draw it, sing it, dance it.

3 MEETING BODY & SOUL

Although split in our materialistic culture, flesh and spirit are linked by the fact that everything, in the language of science, is waves of energy.

So here are some exercises to help you become more aware of the subtle energies of your body, knowing that the energy that circulates within you is also the energy of the universe and that your body itself is distilled energy, worthy of honour and care.

EXERCISES & MEDITATIONS

A FULLY ACCEPTING THE BODY

Take a hand mirror, make yourself private and comfortable and examine yourself in the mirror. Touch yourself gently and in wonder. This is not a masturbation (although you can - later). It is an exploration, a meditation and a celebration; the folds; the form, the opening; the colours, the contours! This is me, this is she!

Take time to reflect on the words used to describe this part of your anatomy. Think how you might have been ashamed of your genitals in the past. Think of personal situations. Think how legions of women over history have been ashamed of their genitals. Think how they have also been the subject of worship in ancient times. Love your yoni, love yourself. Honour your body, honour yourself, honour all women.

B HEALING THE GENITAL DISCONNECT

Lie down in a quiet comfortable private space, it could be your bath, it could be your bed. Play sweet music if you want to.

Lay one hand over your heart and the other gently across your belly with your fingers touching your mound. Close your eyes and take a few deep breaths. Relax, in whatever way you prefer.

Focus your mind and your senses on the heart area under the one hand, and the womb are under the other. Notice sensations on the skin. Then go deeper inside the body. Feel these places as energy.

And in your mind's eye start to connect the energies of heart and genitals – in a loop, in a circle, in a wave. As energy they are all one and all linked. Love this connection between your symbolic seat of love and your symbolic seat of creativity and fecundity.

See it as a stream of energy of light or filament or whatever comes up for you. Now include your head into this wave. Head and heart and genitals – mental, emotional and physical – linked by ... this energy that you are imagining and experiencing. Let this flow of energy include your entire body.

In this gentle space, you can forgive yourself for the unkind body images you have taken on from our culture. Forgive yourself for the times you have not understood this connection. Enjoy the experience.

C **ACCESSING THE ENERGY**

Stand with you knees bent, or kneel on a soft surface and begin to rock your pelvis backwards and forwards vigorously. All the while breathing vigorously with you mouth open and pursed a little, matching the out breath with the forward thrust of your pelvis.

After at least 30 breaths, while tightening your perineum and sexual muscles, take an extra long slow deep breath, pulling up through your belly, your chest, into your nose. Hold it a moment. Sip another miniscule amount of air through your nose, and then As slowly as you can manage, relax everything.

Notice your body sensations and feelings - the tingle of energy racing everywhere, suffusing you.

What do you feel? (Gee, I suspect you have just had a full body orgasm, without any genital stimulation. We call it the orgasm breath.)

Contemplate this energy: is it erotic, is it physical, is it sensuous, is it energetic? Where does the one begin or end?

Circulate it throughout your body. Do it again.

These are beginner exercises that point to meditations of esoteric sexual practices where the focus is on transforming sexual energy into spirit – into love.

But for now you have had a taste of the wholeness, the oneness, erotic and sensuous within yourself; and with that a sense of bliss which is also spiritual before being with your partner, and even if you don't have a partner.

4 MAKING NEW CHOICES

Now link back to your work in Section 1. Review your notes there. Can you see how your core beliefs created ways of being, role models if you like which have influenced your life.

Examine the stereotypes of aging women that you have read. Are you content with these for you? How about reviewing your core beliefs and choosing new images to live by?

A   CHANGING MY CORE BELIEFS

My new vision of sexuality:

_____
_____
_____
_____
_____
_____
_____

Write more on separate sheets if you need to.

My new understanding of menopause: (and if you have already finished, the menopause I wish I had).

_____
_____
_____
_____
_____

136   Towards a Soulful Sexuality

_____
_____
_____

Write more on separate sheets if you need to.

My new images of life as a post menopausal woman:

_____
_____
_____
_____
_____
_____
_____

Write more on separate sheets if you need to.
How do you feel now? Write it, draw it, sing it, dance it, Live IT!

FUTURE FORWARD

Use the next several pages to write about what you've learned in this exploration of your sexuality. Include commitments and action plan for yourself; daily practises, new learning, books to read, workshops to attend, personal psychotherapy, spiritual counselling, coaching,. issues to heal.

_____
_____
_____
_____
_____

Well done, for having had the courage to complete this Workbook. I am sure you understand a whole lot more about yourself now. And feel more alive, energetic and whole.

BIBLIOGRAPHY

Achterberg, Jeanne. *Woman As Healer*: Shambahla Publications, Inc, Boston, Massachusetts, 1991

Adkinson, Robert (ed). *Sacred Sex*: Thames and Hudson, London, 1997

Agonito, Rosemary (ed). *History of Ideas on Woman*: Perigee Books, New York, 1977

Avalon, Arthur (Sir John Woodroffe). *The Serpent Power: The Secrets of Tantric and Shaktic Yoga*: Dover Publications, Inc, New York, 1974 (1919)

Banner, Lois W. *In Full Flower: Aging Women, Power and Sexuality*: Vintage Books, New York, 1992

Bolen, Jean Shinoda, M.D. *Goddesses in Older Women: Archetypes in Women Over Fifty*: Quill, New York, 2001

Camphausen, Rufus C. *The Yoni: Sacred Symbol of Female Creative Power*: Inner Traditions International, Rochester, Vermont, 1996

Chia, Mantak & Chia, Maneewan. *Awaken Healing Energy Through the Tao*: Aurora Press, Santa Fe, New Mexico, 1983

Chia, Mantak & Chia, Maneewan. *Healing Love Through the Tao: Cultivating Female Sexual Energy*: Healing Tao Books, Huntington, New York, 1988

Chia, Mantak & Winn, Michael. *Taoist Secrets of Love: Cultivating Male Sexual Energy*: Aurora Press, Santa Fe, New Mexico, 1984

Chopra, Deepak. *Ageless Body, Timeless Mind: The Quantum Alternative to Growing Old*: Harmony Books, New York, 1993

Cleary, Thomas (ed). *Immortal Sisters: Secrets of Taoist Women*: Shambhala Publications Inc., Boston, Massachusetts, 1989

Douglas, Nik & Slinger, Penny. *Sexual Secrets: The Alchemy of Ecstasy*: Destiny Books, Rochester, Vermont, 1979

Diamant, Anita. *The Red Tent*: Picador, St Martins, 1997

Ellis, Havelock. *Studies in the Psychology of Sex, Volume I*: F.A. Davis Company Publishers, Philadelphia, 1900

Ellis, Havelock. *Studies in the Psychology of Sex, Volume IV*: F.A. Davis Company Publishers, Philadelphia, 1905

Evola, Julius. *Eros and the Mysteries of Love*: Inner Traditions International, Rochester, Vermont, 1969

Freud, Sigmund. *On Sexuality: Three Essays on the Theory of Sexuality, Volume 7*: Penguin Books, Middlesex, England, 1953

Friday, Nancy. *The Power of Beauty*: Hutchinson, London, 1996

Friedan, Betty. *The Feminine Mystique*: Penguin Books, Middlesex, England, 1963

Harding, M. Esther. *Women's Mysteries: Ancient and Modern*: Shambhala Publications Inc. Boston, Massachusetts, 1971

Hollis, James. *Creating a Life: Finding Your Individual Path*, Inner City Books, Toronto, Canada, 2001

Kahn Ladas, Alice, Whipple, Beverly & Perry, John D. *The G Spot and Other Recent Discoveries About Human Sexuality*: Corgi Books, London, 1982

Kinsey, Alfred C. *Sexual Behavior in the Human Female*: W.B. Saunders Company, New York, 1953

Kisch, Heinrich E. *The Sexual Life of Woman in its Physiological and Hygienic Aspect*, Medical Arts Agency, New York, 1931

Krog, Antjie. *Body Bereft*: Umuzi, Johannesburg, 2006

Lai, Hsi. *The Sexual Teachings of the White Tigress: Secrets of the Female Taoist Masters*: Destiny Books, Rochester, Vermont, 2001

Lowen, Alexander. M.D. *The Spirituality of the Body: BioEnergetics for Grace and Harmony*: Macmillan Publishing Company, New York, 1990

Lowndes Sevely, Josephine. *Eve's Secrets: A New Theory of Female Sexuality*: Random House, New York, 1987

Morris, Desmond. *The Naked Woman: A Study of the Female Body*: Vintage Books, London, 2004

Murdock, Maureen. *The Heroine Journey*: Shambhala Publications Inc., Boston, Massachusetts, 1990

Paglia, Camille. *Sexual Personae: Art and Decadence from Nefertiti to Emily Dickinson*: Vintage Books, New York, 1990

Paglia, Camille. *Sex, Art and American Culture*: Penguin Books, London, 1992

Patai, Raphael. *The Hebrew Goddess*: Wayne State University Press, Detroit, Michigan, 1967

Qualls-Corbett, Nancy. *The Sacred Prostitute: Eternal Aspect of the Feminine*: Inner City Books, Toronto, Canada, 1988

Ramsdale, David & Ramsdale, Ellen. *Sexual Energy Ecstasy: A Practical Guide to Lovemaking Secrets of the East and West*: Bantom Books, New York, 1985

Reich, Wilhelm. *The Function of the Orgasm: The Discovery of the Orgone*: Meridian, New York, 1942

Robinson, James M (ed). *The Nag Hammadi Library: The Definitive Translation of the Gnostic Scriptures Complete in One Volume*: HarperSanFrancisco, New York, 1978

Shaw, Miranda. *Passionate Enlightenment: Women In Tantric Buddhism*: Princeton University Press, Princeton, New Jersey, 1994

Silburn, Lilian. *Kundalini Energy of the Depths*: State University of New York Press, Albany, New York, 1988

Tannahill, Reay. *Sex In History*: Abacus, London, 1979

Tunneshende, Merilyn. *Rainbow Serpent: The Magical Art of Sexual Energy*: Thorsons, London, 1999

Walker, Barbara. G. *The Crone: Woman of Age, Wisdom and Power*: HarperSanFrancisco, New York, 1985

Williams, Brandy. *Ecstatic Ritual: Practical Sex Magic*: Prism Press, Great Britain, 1990

Woodman, Marion & Dickson, Elinor. *Dancing in the Flames: The Dark Goddess in the Transformation of*

Consciousness: Shambhala Publications Inc., Boston, Massachusetts, *1997*
Zohar, Danah. *The Quantum Self:* Flamingo, London, *1991*

USEFUL WEBSITES

www.tamboo.co.za
www.birthingthecrone.com

ENDNOTES

1. Robinson, James M (ed). *The Nag Hammadi Library: The Definitive Translation of the Gnostic Scriptures Complete in One Volume:* HarperSanFrancisco, New York, 1978, p. 297. The section called "The Thunder: Perfect Mind" is a revelation discourse by an unidentified ancient female figure. Isis, Eve, and Sophia are suggested, but who can know?
2. Banner, Lois W. *In Full Flower: Aging Women, Power and Sexuality:* Vintage Books, New York, 1992, p. 59.
3. Evola, Julius. *Eros and the Mysteries of Love:* Inner Traditions International, Rochester, Vermont, 1969, p. 56.
4. Degler, Carl. "What Ought to Be and What Was: Women's Sexuality in the Nineteenth Century", American Historical Review, Dec. 1974, p. 1483. Quoted in Lowndes Sevely, Josephine. *Eve's Secrets: A New Theory of Female Sexuality:* Random House, New York, 1987, p. xiii.
5. Ibid. p. xv.
6. Lowen, Alexander, M.D. *The Spirituality of the Body: BioEnergetics for Grace and Harmony:* Macmillan Publishing Company, New York, 1990, p. 103.
7. Friday, Nancy. *The Power of Beauty:* Hutchinson, London, 1996, p. 498.
8. Bolen, Jean Shinoda M.D. *Goddesses in Older Women: Archetypes in Women Over Fifty:* Quill, New York, 2001, Footnote, p. 25.
9. Friday. *The Power of Beauty,* p. 498.
10. Douglas, Nik & Slinger, Penny. *Sexual Secrets: The Alchemy of Ecstasy:* Destiny Books, Rochester, Vermont, 1979, p. 141.
11. For more insight into these theories of age defiance, refer to Deepak Chopra M.D.'s *Ageless Body, Timeless Mind: The Quantum Alternative to Growing Old:* Harmony Books, New York, 1993.
12. "Wonder Woman", Sunday Times (South Africa), 14 May 2006, p. 3.
13. Friday. *The Power of Beauty,* p. 503.
14. Banner. *In Full Flower,* p. 295.
15. Ibid. p. 192
16. Ibid.
17. Ibid.
18. Ibid. p. 189.
19. Witches Hammer, by Heinrich Kramer & Jacob Sprenger, quoted in Banner. p. 191.
20. Banner. *In Full Flower,* p. 191
21. Ibid. p. 194.
22. Ibid. p. 383.
23. Lowndes Sevely. *Eve's Secret,* p. xiii.

24. Ibid.
25. Ibid. p. 277.
26. Banner. In Full Flower, p. 253.
27. Ibid. p. 255.
28. Literary personas of lusty aging women, menacing housekeepers, ageing brothel madams, and midwives-cum-healers coexisted with this idealised middle-class image.
29. Ibid. p. 277.
30. Ibid.
31. Ibid. p. 276.
32. Ibid. p. 281.
33. Ibid. p. 282.
34. Ibid. p. 284.
35. Kisch, Enoch Heinrich. The Sexual Life of Women. Quoted in Banner, In Full Flower, p. 281.
36. Kisch, Enoch Heinrich. The Sexual Life of Women: Medical Art Agency, New York, p. 340. *My emphasis.*
37. Banner. In Full Flower, p. 287.
38. Ibid. p. 280.
39. Ibid. p. 284.
40. Banner. In Full Flower, p. 274.
41. Ibid.
42. Ibid. p. 285.
43. Ibid. p. 240. *(My emphasis.)*
44. Ibid. p. 295.
45. Ibid. p. 274.
46. Ibid. p. 278.
47. Ibid.
48. Wylie, Philip. Generation of Vipers: Rinehart, New York, 1942, pp. 186-187. Quoted in Banner. p. 303.
49. Ibid. p. 291.
50. Ibid. p. 297.
51. Ibid. p. 274.
52. Ibid. p. 299.
53. Ibid. p. 300.
54. Ibid. p. 301.

55. Ibid. p. 300-1.
56. Ibid. p. 304.
57. Erikson, Erik, H. *Childhood and Society:* WW Norton & Company, Inc. USA, 1950, Quoted in Banner. p. 303.
58. Ibid. p. 292.
59. Cleary, Thomas (ed). *Immortal Sisters: Secrets of Taoist Women:* Shambhala Publications Inc., Boston, Massachusetts, 1989, p. 91.
60. Some of these practices involved stopping the flow of menstrual blood during a women's generative prime, in the same way as males stopped the flow of semen. Both stem from a negative view of the body. Nevertheless, the idea of a deliberate and harmonious experience of menopause, whatever that might turn out to be, is profoundly required.
61. Douglas, Nik. et al. *Sexual Secrets,* p. 141
62. Redman, Helen. "Menopause Gallery" found at www.birthingthecrone.com/pages/meno.html.
63. Bolen. *Goddesses in Older Women,* p. xxiv.
64. Krog, Antjie. *Body Bereft:* Umuzi, Johannesburg, 2006, p. 16. This book of poetry by a wonderful South African author includes a searing series of menopause poems.
65. Evola. *Eros and the Mysteries of Love,* p. 150.
66. Lowndes Sevely, Josephine. *Eve's Secrets,* p. 7.
67. Freud, Sigmund. "Woman as Castrated Man," in Agonito, Rosemary (ed). *History of Ideas on Woman:* Perigee Books, New York, 1977, p. 319 (My emphasis.)
68. Friday. *The Power of Beauty.* p. 64.
69. Ibid. p. 494.
70. Paglia, Camille. *Sexual Personae: Art and Decadence From Nefertiti to Emily Dickinson:* Vintage Books, London, 2004, p. 17.
71. Achterberg, Jeanne. *Woman as Healer:* Shambhala, Boston, Massachussetts, p. 86.
72. Camphausen, Rufus C. *The Yoni: Sacred Symbol of Female Creative Power:* Inner Traditions International, Rochester, Vermont, 1996.
73. See www.tamboo.co.za for the work of Mordechai Brodie.
74. Greer, Germaine. *The Madwoman's Underclothes,* Atlantic Monthly Press, New York, 1987, p. 38. Quoted in Friday. *The Power of Beauty.* p. 507.
75. Lowndes Sevely. *Eve's Secrets,* p. xx.
76. Fallopio, Gabriel. *Observationes Anatomicae,* 1561, quoted in Lowndes Sevely. *Eve's Secrets.* p. 12.
77. Ibid. p. 17. The following discussion is based on extracts from Lowndes Sevely's discussion on the male and female genitalia.
78. Ibid. p. 136.333
79. Ibid. p. 139.

80. Evola. *Eros and the Mysteries of Love*, p. 160 My emphasis.
81. Ibid. p. 159.
82. Ibid. p. 160.
83. Ibid. p. 159.
84. Anderson Duana R. *Hysteria: The Wandering Uterus & A Brief History of the Vibrator*, found at www.necrobabes.org/duana/hysteria.html
85. Banner. *In Full Flower*, p. 193.
86. Freud. Sigmund. *On Sexuality: Three Essays on the Theory of Sexuality, Volume 7*: Penguin Books, Middlesex, England, 1953, p. 79. My emphasis.
87. Kinsey, Alfred C. *Sexual Behavior in the Human Female*: W.B. Saunders Company, New York, 1953, p. 362. My emphasis.
88. Morris Desmond. *The Naked Woman: A Study of the Female Body*: Vintage Books, London, 2004, p. 210, 212.
89. Kahn Ladas, Alice, Whipple, Beverly & Perry, John D. *The G Spot and Other Recent Discoveries About Human Sexuality*: Corgi Books, London, 1982, p. 146.
90. Kinsey. *Sexual Behavior in the Human Female*: p. 655.
91. Lowen, Alexander. M.D. *The Spirituality of the Body: BioEnergetics for Grace and Harmony*: Macmilan Publishing Company, New York, 1990, p. 22.
92. Evola. *Eros and the Mysteries of Love*, p. 273.
93. Ibid. p. 17.
94. Ibid. p. 22.
95. Ibid., p. 18.
96. Ramsdale, David & Ramsdale, Ellen. *Sexual Energy Ecstasy: A Practical Guide to Lovemaking Secrets of the East and West*: Bantom Books, New York, 1985, p. 46.
97. Rabbi Nachshon (Nachshon of Breslov). *The Fiftieth Gate*.
98. Evola. *Eros and the Mysteries of Love*, p. 180.
99. Ficino, Marsilio. *Sopra lo amore*, VII; I, 3. Quoted in Evola. *Eros and the Mysteries of Love*, p. 55.
100. Shakespeare, William, *The Complete Works of William Shakespeare*, Oxford Standard Authors edition, Oxford University Press, London: 1959, Sonnet CXXIX. p. 1124.
101. Evola. *Eros and the Mysteries of Love*, p. 273.
102. Ibid. p. 273.
103. Patai, Raphael. *The Hebrew Goddess*: Wayne State University Press, Detroit, Michigan, 1967, p. 177.
104. Evola. *Eros and the Mysteries of Love*, p. 181.
105. See all of the works by Mantak Chia mentioned in the Bibliography.
106. Ibid. p. 85.

107. *Websters Comprehensive Dictionary of the English Language, Encyclopedic Edition:* Trident Press International, Florida, 1996.
108. Evola. *Eros and the Mysteries of Love,* p. 44.
109. Ibid. p. 101.
110. *Job* 19:26.
111. Lowen. *The Spirituality of the Body,* p. 103.
112. *The Columbia Encyclopedia,* Sixth Edition, 2001-2005. The passage quoted describes the neo-Platonic Renaissance theories of Judah Abravanel (Leo the Hebrew), 15th century Jewish philosopher, physician, and poet. See www.bartleby.com/65/ab/Abravan-J.html and http://en.wikipedia.org/wiki/Judah_Leon_Abravanel.
113. Douglas, Nik, et al, *Sexual Secrets,* p. 145.
114. Chia, Mantak & Winn, Michael. Introduction, *Taoist Secrets of Love: Cultivating Male Sexual Energy:* Aurora Press, Santa Fe, New Mexico, 1984, p. iii.
115. Fritjof Capra, *The Tao of Physics,* On Quantum Theory. Quoted in www.spaceandmotion.com/Physics-Quantum-Theory-Mechanics.html.
116. Douglas, Nik, et al. *Sexual Secrets,* p. 131.
117. Zohar, Dana. *The Quantum Self:* William Morrow, 1990, p. 101. Quoted in Woodman, Marion & Dickson, Elinor. *Dancing in the Flames: The Dark Goddess in the Transformation of Consciousness:* Shambhala Publications Inc., Boston, Massachusetts, 1997, p. 210.
118. Robinson. *The Nag Hammadi Library,* p. 302.
119. *The Concise Oxford Dictionary:* Clarendon Press, England, 1990.
120. Bolen. *Goddesses in Older Women,* p. 46.
121. Ibid. p. 156.
122. Walker, Barbara. G. *The Crone: Woman of Age, Wisdom and Power:* HarperSanFrancisco, New York, 1985 , p. 30.
123. Ibid. p. 129.
124. Friday. *The Power of Beauty,* p. 514.
125. Patai, Raphael. *The Hebrew Goddess:* Wayne State University Press, Detroit, Michigan, 1967. For a more comprehensive take on these ideas, please refer to Patai's text.
126. Diamant, Anita. *The Red Tent:* Picador, St Martins, 1997.
127. Walker. *The Crone.*
128. Ibid. p. 59.
129. Woodman, Marion, et al. *Dancing in the Flames,* p. 207.
130. Murdock. *The Heroine's Journey:* Shambahla Publications, Inc. Boston, Massachusetts, 1990, pp. 162-164.
131. Robinson. *The Nag Hammadi Library,* p. 301.

132. Ibid. p. 222.
133. Ibid. p. 49.
134. Woodman, et al. Dancing in the Flames, p. 222.
135. Ibid. p. 211.
136. Hollis, James. Creating a Life: Finding Your Individual Path, Inner City Books, Toronto, Canada, 2001.
137. Friday. The Power of Beauty, p. 499.
138. Ibid. p. 532.
139. Go see Helen Redman's amazing paintings on www.birthingthecrone.com/.
140. Robinson, The Nag Hammadi Library, p. 301.
141. Feminist philosopher Anais Nin on Love.

FURTHER INFORMATION

Adele Gruber, like most people, has worn many masks. These include being mother and grandmother, wife, student, teacher, business woman and professional publisher. Now Adele dedicates herself to her life-long passion in dance, yoga, meditation and body modalities. She has a special interest in the body-mind-soul continuum and in how movement and body awareness affects our life.

This enduring interest has been given intellectual structure and experiential expression through her on-going studies of Archetypal Psychotherapy and the applied consciousness teachings with the Tamboo Academy, run by Mordechai and Siobhan Brodie. Adele also assisted in bringing **Biodanza** to South Africa. Her training includes the range of **Kadeisha** workshops as well as extensive training in Imaginal Psychology. Adele's particular interests include dance as sacred practice, healthy aging, women's mythology and Conscious Sexuality.

Adele runs her original workshop series, called HolyMoves, which provides a experiential format for all women to explore the interface of spirituality and sexuality as it affects body and soul. She practices as an Imaginal therapist and conscious body counselor and lives in Cape Town.

HolyMoves© Workshops provide the safe context and profound processes for adult women to explore their rich, deep capacities as complete, spiritual and sensuous, modern women. It is a precious opportunity to tap into the patterns and potentials of their inner holy places – in a surprising way. It is a gentle, very personal, journey of inspiration, information and entertainment that touches the deeply feminine self and supports a shift of viewing point.

Distilling elements and essential insights from myth, history, archetypal psychology, science, body therapies and eastern (tantric) systems into a potent brew, HolyMoves is an initiatory experience for modern women, engaging these profound mysteries from a holistic, experiential, soul-based perspective. The workshops combine lectures, discussion, movements, meditations and exercises into a wonderful new dance of self.

Please check **www.holymoves.com** for current workshops or contact **adele@gruber.co.za** to schedule workshops in your area.

The Tamboo Academy is an umbrella organisation that covers a wide range of training and practices in physical well-being, sexual health, ecological and personal growth, intimacy and relationships, self-expression and creativity, psychotherapeutic development and spiritual evolution. The insights and practical methods developed in Shamanism, Kabbalah, Alchemy, Tantra and Taoism are all used together with more contemporary wisdom. The formal orientation of Archetypal Psychotherapy is based on C.G. Jung's psychology, as developed further by James Hillman and others.

Please visit **www.tamboo.co.za** for more information.

www.ingramcontent.com/pod-product-compliance
Lightning Source LLC
Chambersburg PA
CBHW051401290426
44108CB00015B/2112